Living with Diverticulitis

A Holistic Four-Phase Diet & Lifestyle Guide To
Manage Flare-Ups, Enhance Gut Health & Well-Being

Prem Nand

Clinical Dietitian – Nutritionist

Copyright © Prem Nand, 2024

All rights reserved. No part of this book may be reproduced or used in any manner without written permission of the copyright owner except for the use of quotations in a book review.

First paperback edition August 2024

Book Format and Cover designed by Cindy Hyde.

Food photography by Jackie Boucher and Ariella Hoko.

For more information, please contact Prem Nand, Maximised Nutrition Ltd (publisher@maximisednutrition.com).

Published Maximised Nutrition Ltd (https://maximisednutrition.com/)

ISBN (standard paperback): 978-1-0670309-2-6
ISBN (premium paperback): 978-1-0670309-3-3
ISBN (kindle e-book): 978-1-0670309-1-9

Dedicated To:

My parents in Fiji: Vinod Kumari Nand and Nitya Nand
&
in the loving memory of my Kiwi parents: Michael & Beverley Deverell

Legal Disclaimer

This dietary and lifestyle guidance with recipes provided in this book are for educational purposes and to support you in your health journey. If you have specific dietary needs or health issues, please consult your physician or a registered dietitian for an individualized plan. For full disclaimer, go to the back page of the book.

PREFACE

Why Is Diverticular Disease An Issue?

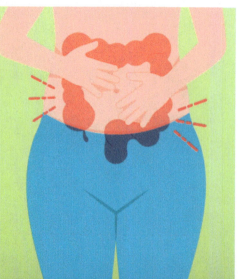

WHY IS DIVERTICULAR DISEASE AN ISSUE?

- Can affect quality of life.
- Those with symptoms can suffer from recurrent pain & discomfort.

25% of those with diverticular disease can develop complications including:

- Abscess (pus in pockets)
- Fistula (irregular passage between bowel and other organs)

Can lead to:

- Tears in the bowel that causes waste to spill out
- Blockages in the bowel
- Hospitalisation and surgery

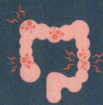

©Maximised Nutrition Ltd

Why Is A Holistic & Comprehensive Management Pathway Needed For Diverticular Disease?

Answer: This has to do with the current classification of diverticular disease.

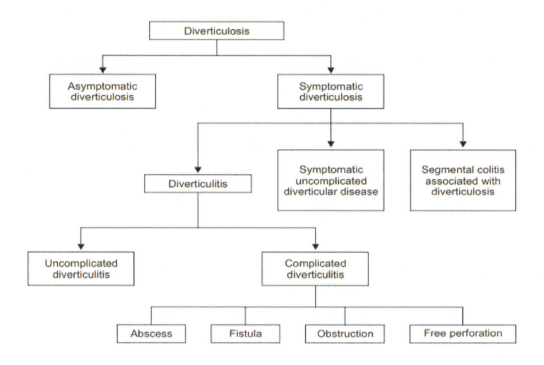

Image from Update on Pathogenesis and Management 2018

You can see from this classification flow chart the various branches of diverticular disease. Thus, the actual flare-up called diverticulitis is just one manifestation of the diverticular disease.

Reference: Rezapour, M., et al. (2018). Diverticular disease: An update on pathogenesis and management. *Gut and Liver*, 12(2), 125-132

Check If You Have Any of These Symptoms of Diverticular Disease

Note, some of these symptoms can be related to other medical conditions such as Inflammatory Bowel Disease, Coeliac Disease, Irritable Bowel Syndrome or even Bowel Cancer.

It is crucial to get timely medical intervention if any of these symptoms persist.

1. **Diverticulosis (usually symptom-free, but some people may notice the following):**

   - Mild cramps or a bit of discomfort in your abdomen
   - Feeling bloated or having a lot of gas
   - Changes in how often you go to the bathroom, either constipation or diarrhoea
   - Sometimes passing mucus when you go to the toilet
   - Mild pain, typically on the lower left side of your belly
   - Feeling like you have not fully emptied your bowels

2. **Diverticulitis (when the diverticula get inflamed or infected):**

   - Sharp, intense pain, often in the lower left part of your abdomen
   - Fever, sometimes with chills
   - Nausea or throwing up
   - Constipation, but sometimes diarrhoea instead
   - Your belly may feel tender or swollen
   - In some cases, there might be blood in your stool or bleeding from the rectum

3. **Symptomatic Uncomplicated Diverticular Disease (SUDD) (ongoing chronic unwellness)**

   - Ongoing pain, often on the lower left side of your abdomen
   - Bloating or feeling full and distended
   - Alternating between being constipated and having diarrhoea
   - Mucus in your stool
   - Feeling like you did not finish going to the bathroom
   - General discomfort, especially after eating

The symptoms of SUDD can be misdiagnosed as those of Irritable Bowel Syndrome.

4. **Diverticular Disease with SIBO/IMO (Small Intestinal Bacterial Overgrowth or Intestinal Methanogen Overgrowth):**

- A lot of bloating and gas, especially after meals and especially after having a carbohydrate food.
- Chronic diarrhoea, or sometimes switching between diarrhoea and constipation
- Excessive burping or passing gas
- Feeling tired or having difficulty concentrating (often referred to as "brain fog")
- Symptoms related to poor nutrient absorption, like losing weight or having deficiencies
- Abdominal pain or discomfort that tends to get worse after you eat

The symptoms can overlap and might vary in how severe they are, depending on the stage and type of diverticular disease. The symptoms can overlap and might vary in how severe they are, depending on the stage and type of diverticular disease. Sometimes, the symptoms of SUDD and SIBO/IMO related to diverticular disease can be misdiagnosed as Irritable Bowel Syndrome.

Track your symptoms and use the guidelines in this book to get an appropriate treatment as needed. If you have any bleeding, Consult with your GP, or Specialist.

Symptom Checklist

SYMPTOM	Tick to indicate symptom is present	Any other comments
Discomfort in abdomen - Mild - Sharp, intense pain - On-going pain		
Feeling Bloated, with gas		
Changes to how often you go to toilet - Constipation or - Diarrhoea or - Both		
Feeling nausea or throwing up		
Passing of mucus when going to toilet		
Feeling that you have not emptied your bowels fully		
Fever, sometimes with chills		
Belly is tender or swollen		
Blood in stool		
Discomfort after eating		
Definite bloating after eating carbohydrate containing food, like bread or pasta or potato or rice		
Excessive burping of passing of wind		
Feeling tired or difficulty concentrating ("foggy brain")		
Losing weight		
Nutrient deficiencies e.g. iron deficiency		
Passing of excessive wind - Flatulence stink		

Symptom Monitoring Tool

Date	Your Symptoms	What you did & what happened

Learn about Diverticulitis

Diverticulitis is an inflammation process that involves the Diverticular (pockets that form in the colon). The number of diverticular increases with age. Acute Diverticulitis can be complicated or uncomplicated.

This book will:

- help you understand the different categories of diverticular disease & their symptoms.

- teach you how to manage diverticulitis flare-ups and symptoms through diet and lifestyle through a four (4) stage management plan.

- guide you to manage each type of diverticular disease with the right diet & lifestyle plan for each stage, even when to seek help from your health care professional.

- help you adapt your everyday meals for a diverticulitis episode.
-
    discuss what to eat and what supplements to use to meet your recommended daily intake/allowance for nutrients.

- give you access to a 21-day menu with delicious recipes to manage stage three of your management plan.

- These menus are professionally designed and nutritionally analyzed with recommendations for portion control for meals and snacks to meet recommended daily nutrient requirements by age and gender categories for those living in Australia, New Zealand & the United States of America.

- guide you about diet & lifestyle management post-acute diverticulitis.

- Share how a particular category of diverticular can be misdiagnosed as Irritable Bowel Syndrome (IBS) and how to nutritionally manage it.

- discuss a holistic healthy eating & lifestyle guide to have during the well stage of this disease.

Holistic & Comprehensive Diet & Lifestyle Solution To Diverticular Disease

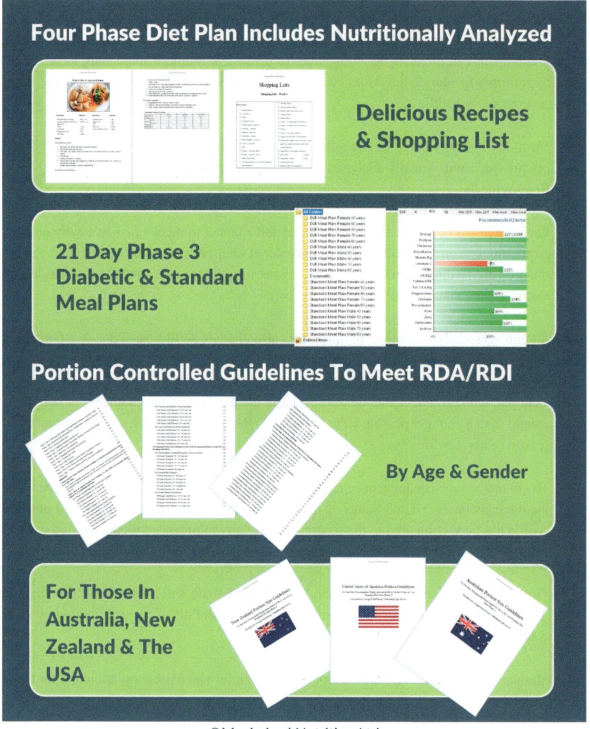

©Maximised Nutrition Ltd

What's Unique About This Nutrition Education Book?

- Most diverticulitis management plan provide a 3-stage management option. My clinical experience with patients shows that a four-stage management plan is a better option, so that patients can fluctuate between stages as needed. With the 4-stage plan, there is an opportunity to address the issues causing diverticulitis / diverticular disease to prevent recurrence, hopefully.

- Most diet information gives you a list of allowed foods and not allowed foods but does not provide a nutritionally analyzed plan that meets your Recommended Daily Requirements.

- Each menu has been nutritionally analyzed and adapted to meet a person's daily nutrient requirement. You may feel unwell in one part of your body, but you need to make sure that you are feeding the rest of your body what it needs for maximum health. These menus ensure that you are.

- As one ages, daily nutritional requirements also change. A 40-year-old active female's nutritional needs are different from those of a 70-year-old sedentary female. It is the same for males. Each decade can mean significant changes in nutritional requirements. For example, with protein, someone over 70 has a greater protein requirement per body weight than a younger person. Hence, what he /she eats needs to be adapted for that season of his /her life.

- The menu and recipes have been analyzed using country-specific nutritional values for the three countries: United States of America, Australia, and New Zealand. The nutrient profile has been compared to the recommended daily allowance / intake for that specific country and its population and against nutrient requirements for age/gender categories.

  Thus, the menu plan for an Australian 55-year-old female will be different from that of an American 55-year-old female. The information and meal plans can still be used by other countries.

- Menu and supplement recommendations are given for standard population and for those with Diabetes.

Other Unique Features have not been listed above. There are many gold nuggets given within each chapter of the book to provide the most comprehensive dietary management plan.

The Importance of Meeting Recommended Dietary Allowances / Intakes (RDAs/RDIs) Through The Menu

The recipes that accompany the 21 Day Menu (both for Standard Population and for those with Diabetes) have been developed as part of the mean plan for the day to meet the RDAs / RDIs for the day.

What does this mean?

Understanding Recommended Dietary Allowance/Intakes

The graph below shows the distribution of a population according to the amount of nutrient they eat on daily basis.

In the graph below, it is seen that 50% of the population will require less than the Estimated Average Requirement (EAR) and 50% will require more than the EAR to meet their individual nutrient requirement for the day.

Regarding the USA population, Food and Drug Administration has determined that 97.5% of the population will meet their daily requirements for the nutrient if they eat the level of nutrients recommended by the FDA (known as Recommended Dietary Allowances or RDAs).

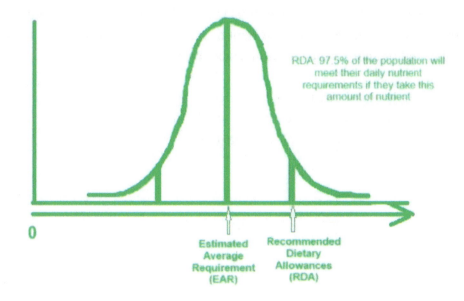

Similarly, the Ministry of Health for Australia and New Zealand have set the Recommended Dietary Intakes (RDIs) levels to meet 97% to 98% of the population's daily nutrient needs if the population eats food meeting these levels.

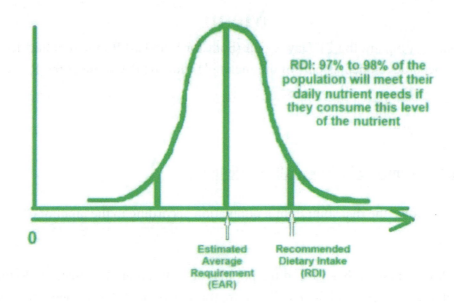

Note, that these levels are recommended for the healthy population.

Gut issues can affect nutrient absorption. That means not all nutrients may be absorbed.

With Low Roughage Diet (Phase 3 of this plan), since whole grain foods, legumes, food containing lot of insoluble fibers are limited (thus potentially affecting level of zinc, manganese, magnesium, selenium, Vitamin Bs) it is important that a meal plan meets at least the RDAs for nutrients with diet and/or appropriate nutritional supplements.

Always be aware of how your body responds to each stage of the diverticular management plan. Watch your energy levels and your bowel motion and food intake. If needed for an individualized nutritional plan, see a qualified nutritionist, naturopath or a registered dietitian.

Case Studies

Case Study 1

A male in his early 60s' European came to the clinic with the following symptoms: extremely fatigued, depressed, lack of sleep, and ongoing abdominal pain. He stated that he had ongoing bloody diarrhea - 3 to 4 times a day. He had been to his GP but was told that it was related to hemorrhoids. He had previously had a hemorrhoidectomy for the same reason, but this had not stopped the bleeding. He stated that he had been eating whatever he could but recently had been too afraid to eat due to pain and bleeding.

Further questioning by Prem Nand, Clinical Dietitian and Nutritionist, showed that he had been diagnosed with diverticular disease five years ago. Prem Nand decided that his symptoms were related likely to diverticulitis flare-up.

Prem Nand wrote to the GP requesting a review of this client regarding a possible diverticulitis flare-up and suggesting that the GP consider an antibiotic. Unfortunately, the locum GP declined to review the client as he felt this was related to his hemorrhoids.

Prem Nand then took this client through phase 2 of the five-step guide, ensuring that his bowel got the rest it needed but ensuring complete nutritional intake. Within four days, the Client stated that the bleeding had stopped, and he only went to empty his bowel twice a day. Prem recommended he stay on phase 2 for a week and then start introducing some food as per phase 3 of the program. Over a month, the Client stated that he had better energy levels, his bowel motions were now formed, and while he did have a couple of episodes of blood streaks on his toilet paper, this had improved. His abdominal pain had subsided, so he was sleeping better. Prem Nand also introduced the right probiotic (discussed within this program). The client also stated that his mental health was a lot better.

Case Study 2

An Asian woman in her mid-50s self-referred to the clinic with IBS symptoms. She had done her research on IBS and had tried to implement information to help with the symptoms. She found Prem Nand, Clinical Dietitian - Nutritionist on the search engine.

On reviewing this client, Prem Nand found that she had also been diagnosed a few years ago with diverticular disease through a colonoscopy. Prem Nand felt that her symptoms were more part of "Symptomatic Uncomplicated Diverticular Disease (SUDD)," which had similar symptoms to IBS. Thus, Prem Nand was able to provide the right advice to this client on how to manage her symptoms.

Case Study 3

Female in mid-60s, post-menopausal, with Obesity Level 2, depression, and fatigue. She came to the clinic to get a diet that could help her lose weight and increase her energy. On assessment, it was found that she had non-insulin-dependent diabetes and ongoing, intermittent bowel pain with diarrhea. She had been told after a colonoscopy many years ago that she had mild diverticular disease.

Her nutrition plan was two-fold:

1) Prem Nand, Clinical Dietitian-Nutritionist, believed that diarrhea and pain occurred during an episode of diverticulitis. Therefore, she wrote a plan for resting her bowel and following a low-roughage diabetic diet.

2) For a well state, Prem Nand designed a low-GI meal plan that included nutritional supplements to help her bowel heal and improve her bowel microbiota.

Six weeks' follow-up showed that her energy levels were better. While she did not lose significant weight, her bowel motions were now regular and soft-formed, and her mood was better. She stated waking up one morning with this mental clarity and energy. Prem Nand reminded her to pace her activities to allow her body to recover.

Case Study 4

An elderly man in his early 80s with bowel incontinence, general body pain, fatigue, and depression. Assessment showed that he had been diagnosed with diverticular disease in his 60s, but no information had been given to him. He had been charted lactulose / laxsol for bowel management and told to be on a high-fiber diet.

Prem Nand, Clinical Dietitian-Nutritionist, was of the view that it was likely that his general body pain was related to demyelination of his nerves. A blood test for homocysteine level confirmed that he was likely under myelinating.

Prem placed this client on a dairy-free diet with phase 3 of this nutrition management plan. She also provided advice on probiotics and relevant nutritional supplements to help myelinate his nerves.

It took a few weeks for his bowel motions to become formed and soft. It took approximately three months for the client to notice a significant improvement in his general body pain. He also noted that he could do a little more around the house. He indicated some improvement in the level of depression he had.

Prem Nand has seen firsthand how these dietary adjustments can make a significant difference. For example, a patient misdiagnosed with IBS found relief by following a diet tailored to management of diverticular disease (that had the category of Symptomatic Uncomplicated Diverticular Disease (SUDD)).

This book helps you better understand your condition and how to manage it. By making informed dietary choices and understanding the underlying mechanisms of diverticular disease, you can improve your quality of life. Always consult your healthcare provider before making significant changes to your diet or treatment plan.

The field of diverticular disease management is evolving, and staying informed about the latest research and treatment options is crucial. With the right approach, including the use of prebiotics, probiotics, and tailored dietary plans, you can effectively manage your diverticular disease and reduce the frequency and severity of symptoms. Remember, the goal is not only to manage your condition but also to enhance your overall well-being. Thank you for taking the time to read this, and I hope you find these insights helpful in managing your condition. Take care and best of health!

About the Author

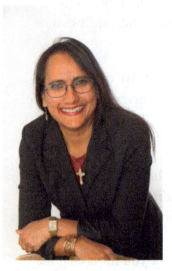

Prem Nand is a Clinical Dietitian and Nutritionist with over 20 years of experience in clinical nutrition and food service menu development. She offers consultancy services to private clients and institutions, having previously worked as a Food Service Dietitian for a regional health board. In this role, Prem developed recipes and menus for over 30 diet codes, ensuring that patients met their nutritional requirements for various medical conditions.

Her personal health journey, including recovery from a car accident and fertility challenges, fuels her passion for understanding human health and wellness. This experience drives her commitment to empowering others in their own health journeys.

Prem also holds a Diploma in Theology and resides in Whangarei, New Zealand.

Prem loves public speaking and is also involved as a leader at Girls Brigade, New Zealand.

Outside of her professional life, she enjoys her extended whanau (family & friends), fishing, gardening, and creating adventures with her daughter, embracing life as it unfolds.

Verified Google Reviews About Prem Nand's Clinical Expertise

Chevaun Nel

★★★★★

I would highly recommend Prem, she has been instrumental in helping me get my health back on track!! I have a complicated medical history and there is no one size fits all with Prem she manages to tailor a plan best suited and individual to you. She has so much knowledge and experience and her advice and support has been invaluable to me. If you are looking to make positive changes in your life or have complicated medical issues you need help with, you have found the perfect person to get you started on a plan that will work for you..... and she is so lovely to work with. Thank you for everything Prem.

Carlysle Vivian-Robins

★★★★★

I've been working with Prem at Maximised Nutrition for a few months and would thoroughly recommend her to anybody with gut-health issues. In my initial consultation I think we both burst in to tears – mine were of total relief and joy that I was at last being heard and taken seriously after several months of symptoms including constant diarrohea, bloating, fatigue and nausea at the mere thought of food. Prem was the first person to take me seriously and shed some light on what was happening in my body and to help me work out a way forward to regaining my health. She explained everything in easy to understand terms and supported me every step of the way, making sure any changes were easily manageable within my limited budget. Her knowledge and skill are equalled by her continual thirst for new research in this area and her genuine passion for seeing people improve their quality of life.

"Hopefully, these reviews show the level of clinical expertise I bring to my practice and what I am putting into this holistic diet and lifestyle management of diverticular disease."

Prem Nand

Clinical Dietitian – Nutritionist, NZRD

Table of Contents

PREFACE

Why Is Diverticular Disease An Issue?

Why Is A Holistic & Comprehensive Management Pathway Needed For Diverticular Disease?

Check If You Have Any of These Symptoms of Diverticular Disease

Symptom Checklist

Symptom Monitoring Tool

Learn about Diverticulitis

Holistic & Comprehensive Diet & Lifestyle Solution To Diverticular Disease

What's Unique About This Nutrition Education Book?

The Importance of Meeting Recommended Dietary Allowances / Intakes (RDAs/RDIs) Through The Menu

Case Studies

About the Author

Verified Google Reviews About Prem Nand's Clinical Expertise

SECTION ONE	1
Chapter 1: Understanding and Managing Diverticulitis	2
Chapter 2: Dietary Phases for Management Of Diverticulitis	10
Chapter 3: Understanding and Implementing Fluid Diets	12
Chapter 4: 19Adapting Recipes for a Low Roughage Diet	19
Chapter 5: Introduction to the 21-Day Low Roughage Menu	26
Chapter 6: Understanding and Managing Symptomatic Uncomplicated Diverticular Disease (SUDD)	29
Chapter 7: Development of SIBO/IMO in Diverticular Disease	34
Chapter 8: Preventing Diverticulitis: Strategies and Tips	36
SECTION TWO	41
21 Day Standard and Diabetic Menus and Shopping Lists	41
Standard Population	42
Diabetic Population	45

Shopping Lists	48
SECTION THREE	56
Recipes	56
Fruit Juice Recipes	57
Smoothie Recipes	59
Soup Recipes	61
Adaptations For Vegan Diet	68
Dinner Recipes	69
SECTION 4	
Country Specific, Gender Specific, Portion Guidelines To Meet Recommended Daily Allowance (USA) or Recommended Dietary Intake (Aust, NZ) For The 21 Day Low Roughage Menu (Phase 3)	111
United States of America Guidelines	112
USA Female (Standard)	113
USA Male (Standard)	114
USA Female (with Diabetes)	115
USA Male (with Diabetes)	116
New Zealand Guidelines	117
NZ Female (Standard)	118
NZ Male (Standard)	119
NZ Female (with Diabetes)	120
NZ Male (with Diabetes)	121
Australian Guidelines	122
Australian Female (Standard)	123
Australian Male (Standard)	124
Australian Female (with Diabetes)	125
Australian Male (with Diabetes)	126
Feedback	127
Legal Disclaimer	127

SECTION ONE

Chapter 1
Understanding and Managing Diverticulitis

Welcome to this comprehensive guide on understanding and managing diverticulitis. Diverticulitis is a condition where pouches called diverticula form in the wall of the intestine, often leading to discomfort and other symptoms. This chapter provides detailed information about diverticulitis, its causes, classifications, and various management strategies. Whether newly diagnosed or looking to manage your condition better, this guide will offer valuable insights into effective dietary and medical interventions.

What is Diverticulitis?

A diverticulum is a pouch that forms when the inner layer of the intestine pushes outward through a weakened part of the digestive tract's wall. This usually happens in the lower part of the large intestine. In a small part of the population, diverticula can develop in the esophagus (gullet).

Here are some terms used regarding this medical condition (Schulz et al., 2020):

Diverticula: The pouch that forms in the colon.

Diverticulosis: The presence of diverticula.

Diverticulitis: When the diverticula become inflamed (about 10 to 25% of those with diverticulosis will experience an inflammation episode in their lifetime).

Diverticular Disease: Any condition involving diverticula, whether symptomatic or asymptomatic.

DIVERTICULOSIS and DIVERTICULITIS

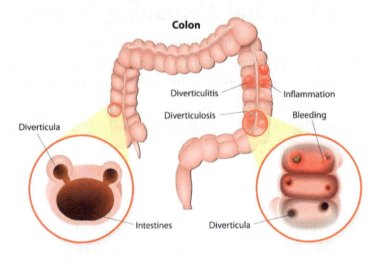

Image purchased from iStock

Classification of Diverticula Disease

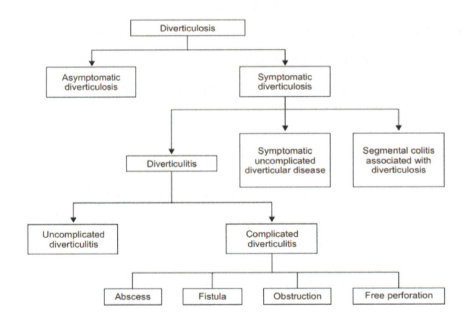

Image from Update on Pathogenesis and Management 2018 (2)

Diverticula starts forming at age 40 in both men and women. Around 10% of the population will have diverticula by the age of 40, but this increases to 50% to 70% in those over 80.

From the diagram above, if someone has diverticulosis, that they may not have any symptoms. However, around 10% to 25% of those with diverticulosis will develop diverticulitis (inflamed diverticula).

Causes of Diverticular Disease

There are many theories about the causes of diverticular disease. Here are a few:

Microbiota Involvement

Our gut has many groups of organisms living in it, including bacteria (both healthy ones and unhealthy ones), viruses, yeast, and archaea. These make up what we call "the Gut Microbiome."

These groups of organisms mostly thrive in harmony with each other. However, when there is an imbalance between them, called dysbiosis, some of the inflammation-producing organisms can increase in their population size.

The products they produce can lead to both inflammation of the bowel surfaces, resulting in certain immune reactions and affecting the nerves in the surface of the intestinal wall. It is thought that this imbalance can lead to the development of diverticula (Rezapour et al., 2018). Research has shown that the bacterial composition around the diverticula is different from the surface of the colon that does not have diverticula in the colon of patients (Schieffer et al., 2017). There are two lines of thought with this discovery: that something is happening to certain gut surfaces that cause the development of diverticula or that having diverticula allows certain bacteria to grow in that area (Schieffer et al., 2017).

"I am of the view that those that end up with diverticulitis likely have poor gut microbiome balance. This may lead to a) some nasty ones living in pockets of your intestine and b) your gut not being able to move properly to remove waste products (called impaired gut motility). The first condition can lead to inflammation and weakening of the gut barrier; the second factor causing pressure to build up in the intestine. The two factors combined then lead to the pressure causing the development of diverticular pockets." (Prem Nand, June 2024). Refer to chapter 6 in this book to learn about the possible role of a leaky gut in diverticulitis.

Low-Fiber Diet

A low-fiber diet can lead to an imbalance in gut microbiota, favoring bacteria that produce inflammatory substances over those that produce anti-inflammatory compounds. However, this is being challenged now by three new studies which indicated that those on a high-fiber diet may have a greater chance of developing diverticulitis (Peery et al., 2012; Yamada et al., 2015;

Braunschmid et al., 2015). This does not mean that we need to have a low-fiber diet but it means that there may be other factors involved in the development of diverticula.

High Body Mass Index (BMI)

A higher BMI, waist-to-hip ratio, or waist circumference is associated with a higher incidence of diverticular disease (Braunschmid et al., 2015).

Smoking

Smokers have higher rates of diverticular disease (Schluz et al., 2020).

High Red Meat Intake

Diets high in red meat increase the risk of diverticular disease (Peery et al., 2012).

Certain Drugs

Medications such as aspirin, NSAIDs, corticosteroids, and opiates can contribute to the development of diverticula (National Institute for Health and Care Excellence [NICE], 2019).

Nerve Changes Related to Aging

As we age, the nerves around the intestine may degenerate. This can lead to altered movements of the bowel, resulting in constipation and increased pressure in the bowel, leading to the development of diverticulitis (Böttner et al., 2013).

How Is Diverticular Disease Diagnosed?

When diagnosing and managing conditions related to the large intestine, such as diverticular disease, doctors use a variety of tests to get a comprehensive understanding of the patient's health. These tests help identify inflammation, blockages, abnormal growths, and other complications. Here are the common diagnostic procedures a doctor might recommend, listed in the typical order they are performed. Your healthcare provider will look at your past health and do a physical exam. They may also use some of the following tests (NICE, 2019):

Flexible Sigmoidoscopy
This test examines the inside part of the large intestine to identify the cause of constipation and other symptoms. A short, flexible, lighted tube with a tiny camera (sigmoidoscope) is inserted through the rectum into the intestine. Air is blown into the intestine to expand it, making it easier to see the intestinal lining. A tissue sample (biopsy) can be taken if necessary.

Barium Enema
Also known as a lower GI (gastrointestinal) series, this X-ray exam visualizes the rectum, large intestine, and the lower part of the small intestine. A metallic fluid called barium is administered as an enema through a tube inserted into the rectum. The barium coats the organs, making them visible on the X-ray, which can then show any narrowed areas (strictures), blockages, or other issues.

Colonoscopy
This procedure inspects the entire length of the large intestine. It can detect abnormal growths, red or swollen tissue, sores (ulcers), or bleeding. A long, flexible, lighted tube with a camera (colonoscope) is inserted through the rectum and advanced into the colon. This allows the healthcare provider to view the colon's lining and take tissue samples (biopsies) if needed, as well as treat certain issues found during the examination.

Virtual Colonoscopy
This procedure involves a CT scan of the colon using air and contrast material. It creates detailed images of the colon to check for polyps, tumors, and other abnormalities without requiring a traditional colonoscopy.

CT Scan
This imaging test provides detailed pictures of various parts of the body, including bones, muscles, fat, and organs. It is used to detect complications of diverticular disease, such as diverticulitis, by revealing inflammation, abscesses, or perforations in the intestines.

These diagnostic tests are crucial in providing a clear and accurate diagnosis, allowing for appropriate and timely treatment of intestinal issues. By following this sequence, doctors can efficiently narrow down the cause of symptoms and identify any complications, ensuring the best possible care for the patient.

Management of Diverticulitis

Diverticulitis, a condition characterized by the inflammation or infection of the diverticula in the digestive tract, requires tailored management strategies depending on the severity of the case. Treatment approaches range from outpatient care for mild cases to hospitalization and surgery for more severe complications. Here are the various management strategies for diverticulitis (NICE, 2019; Severi et al., 2018):

Outpatient Management
For cases without significant complications, diverticulitis can often be managed on an outpatient basis. This may sometimes be done without the need for antibiotics. Dietary adjustments, such as consuming clear fluids and following a low-roughage diet, can help alleviate symptoms, and

promote healing. Patients are typically monitored closely to ensure that their condition does not worsen.

Hospitalization for Small Abscesses

If a patient develops a small abscess (less than one centimeter), hospitalization may be necessary. Treatment involves bowel rest, parenteral fluids, and systemic antibiotics to control the infection. Close monitoring is essential to prevent the abscess from enlarging or causing further complications.

Hospitalization for Larger Abscesses

Larger abscesses (greater than one centimeter) require more intensive treatment, including hospitalization, bowel rest, IV fluids, and systemic antibiotics. In many cases, ultrasound-guided drainage of the abscess is necessary to remove the pus and reduce infection. If the condition is severe or does not respond to these treatments' surgery may be considered to remove the affected portion of the intestine.

Perforation and Peritonitis

In cases of perforation, where the diverticula bursts and pus and inflammation spread throughout the abdominal cavity, immediate hospitalization is critical. Treatment includes bowel rest, IV fluids, and broad-spectrum antibiotics to control the infection. Surgery is typically required to repair the perforation and clean the abdominal cavity to prevent or treat peritonitis, a potentially life-threatening condition.

Effective management of diverticulitis depends on the severity of the condition and timely intervention. Outpatient care can be sufficient for mild cases, while hospitalization and more aggressive treatments are necessary for complications such as abscesses, perforation, and peritonitis. By following these tailored approaches, healthcare providers can ensure the best possible outcomes for patients with diverticulitis.

Possible Complications of Diverticular Disease

Diverticular disease and related intestinal conditions can lead to a range of serious complications, each with distinct symptoms and treatment requirements. Understanding these potential issues is crucial for timely and effective medical intervention. Here are some of the common complications associated with diverticular disease and other intestinal conditions:

Possible complications include:

Holes, Ruptures, or Tears in the Intestines

These can occur due to severe inflammation or injury, leading to the formation of abscesses (sores) or a widespread infection in the abdominal cavity (peritonitis). Peritonitis is a serious condition that can be fatal if not treated promptly.

Infection (Diverticulitis)

This occurs when one or more of the small pouches (diverticula) in the digestive tract become inflamed or infected. Symptoms may include severe abdominal pain, fever, and changes in bowel habits.

Intestinal Blockages

Blockages can happen when the passage of contents through the intestines is obstructed. This can lead to severe abdominal pain, vomiting, and an inability to pass stool or gas. Prompt medical attention is necessary to avoid complications.

Bleeding (Diverticular Bleeding)

This refers to bleeding from a diverticulum, a small bulging pouch in the colon. It can cause bright red or maroon-colored blood in the stool and may require medical intervention to stop the bleeding.

Colitis (Inflammation of the Colon)

This condition involves inflammation of the inner lining of the colon and can result from infections, inflammatory bowel disease, or other conditions. Symptoms include diarrhea, abdominal pain, and sometimes blood in the stool.

Recognizing the signs and symptoms of these complications is essential for early diagnosis and effective treatment. Each condition presents unique challenges, but with prompt medical care, many of these issues can be managed successfully, reducing the risk of severe outcomes. Awareness and understanding of these complications can significantly improve patient prognosis and quality of life.

References

Böttner, M., Barrenschee, M., Hellwig, I., Harde, J., Egberts, J. H., Becker, T., et al. (2013). The GDNF system is altered in diverticular disease – Implications for pathogenesis. *PLoS One*, 8, e66290.

Braunschmid, T., Stift, A., Mittlböck, M., Lord, A., Weiser, F. A., & Riss, S. (2015). Constipation is not associated with diverticular disease – Analysis of 976 patients. *International Journal of Surgery*, 19, 42-45.

Jeganathan, N. A., et al. (2021). The microbiome of diverticulitis. *JGH Open*, Retrieved from https://www.sciencedirect.com/science/article/abs/pii/S2468867321000778

Prem Nand, June 2024: My explanatory comment in this book.

National Institute for Health and Care Excellence (NICE). (2019). Diverticular disease: Diagnosis and management. Retrieved from https://www.nice.org.uk/guidance/ng147

Onur, M. R., et al. (2017). Diverticulitis: A comprehensive review with usual and unusual complications. *Insights into Imaging*, 8(1), 19-27.

Peery, A. F., Barrett, P. R., Park, D., Rogers, A. J., Galanko, J. A., Martin, C. F., et al. (2012). A high-fiber diet does not protect against asymptomatic diverticulosis. *Gastroenterology*, 142, 266-272.

Rezapour, M., et al. (2018). Diverticular disease: An update on pathogenesis and management. *Gut and Liver*, 12(2), 125-132.

Schieffer, K. M., et al. (2017). The microbial ecosystem distinguishes chronically diseased tissue from adjacent tissue in the sigmoid colon of chronic, recurrent diverticulitis patients. *Microbiome*, Retrieved from https://www.ncbi.nlm.nih.gov/pmc/articles/PMC5559482

Schluz, J. K., et al. (2020). European Society of Coloproctology: guidelines for the management of diverticular disease of the colon. *Colorectal Disease*, 22(Suppl 2), 5-28. https://doi.org/10.1111/codi.15140

Severi, C., et al. (2018). Recent advances in understanding and managing diverticulitis. *F1000Research*, 7(F1000 Faculty Rev), 971. https://doi.org/10.12688/f1000research.14091.1

Yamada, E., Inamori, M., Watanabe, S., Sato, T., Tagri, M., Uchida, E., et al. (2015). Constipation is not associated with colonic diverticula: A multicenter study in Japan. *Neurogastroenterology & Motility*, 27, 333-338.

Chapter 2
Dietary Phases for Management Of Diverticulitis

This diet and lifestyle management plan includes a four-stage plan as given below.

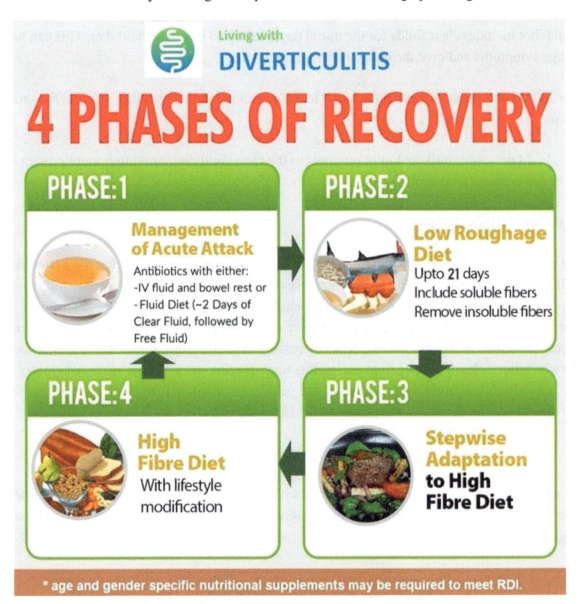

Image designed by Prem Nand, Maximised Nutrition

Phase One: Acute Management, Including The Use Of Fluid Diet

Acute management includes bowel rest with either IV fluid or a fluid diet and possibly outpatient clinic management with or without antibiotics. Severe cases may require bowel rest, IV fluids, parenteral nutrition (feeding through a tube into your vein), and surgery.

A fluid diet includes clear fluids for the initial days, followed by a free fluid diet. This can help manage symptoms and give the gastrointestinal tract a rest.

Clear Fluid Diet: Includes clear liquids that leave no residue in the intestine. Suitable for short-term use.

Free Fluid Diet: Adds milk and milk products to the clear fluid diet, providing more protein but still insufficient for long-term nutrition.

Herxheimer (Herx) Response

Note that for some patients, there will be a Herxheimer response: an acute response between a few hours to 48 hours of starting an antibiotic treatment. The reactions can have the following symptoms: headache, fatigue, tiredness, fever, chills, hyperventilation. It is thought as the bacteria is broken down, they release a substance called lipoprotein, which when absorbed into the body, can lead to an immune response (increasing inflammation). It is important to drink plenty of water / clear liquid or fluid during this time. Having extra Vitamin C may help: try clear juices like clear orange juice. Resting and getting good amounts of sleep is important too. If your blood pressure drops too low, seek medical help urgently.

Phase Two: Low Roughage Diet

This phase requires a low-roughage diet for up to 21 days, focusing primarily on soluble fiber while avoiding rough and insoluble fibers. To assist with this, the book includes a 21-day Low Roughage Menu in Section 2.

Phase Three: Transition to High-Fiber Diet

After the low-roughage phase, gradually introduce a high-fiber diet. Chewing thoroughly is crucial during this transition to ensure proper digestion and prevent discomfort.

This chapter offers valuable insights into managing diverticulitis by understanding its causes, classifications, and dietary management. Following the recommended clear and fluid diets, and eventually transitioning to a high-fiber diet, can provide the necessary support for your gastrointestinal tract during and after an acute attack.

Phase Four: High fiber Diet

This phase of the diet is nutritionally balanced and includes adequate amounts of fiber, healthy fats, proteins, and starchy carbohydrates. I particularly enjoy following the Mediterranean Diet lifestyle, which will be explained in detail later in the book.

Always consult your GP for personalized advice and guidance. By making informed dietary choices and understanding the underlying mechanisms of diverticulitis, you can effectively manage your condition and improve your quality of life. Thank you for reading this chapter. I wish you the best in your journey toward better health and well-being. Take care and stay proactive in managing your health.

Chapter 3
Understanding and Implementing Fluid Diets

Managing diverticulitis involves several steps, and understanding these phases is crucial for effective treatment. We have divided the management process into four distinct phases:

1. Management of an acute attack by resting the bowel using a fluid diet with or without use of antibiotic.
2. Low roughage diet.
3. Stepwise adaptation to a high-fiber diet.
4. Eventually, a full high-fiber diet.

This chapter will focus on the first step: the fluid diet. Understanding and implementing clear and free-fluid diets can help give your gastrointestinal tract the rest it needs during an acute diverticulitis attack. Let us dive into the specifics of these diets and how they can benefit your health.

The fluid diet consists of a clear fluid diet and a free fluid diet.

Clear Fluid Diet

A clear fluid diet includes fluids that are clear and leave no residue in the intestine after digestion. Everything in a clear, fluid diet needs to be absorbed during the digestive process.

Although there is no fiber, the diet should meet the daily nutrient requirement for all nutrients except fiber.

When is a Clear Fluid Diet Used?

A clear fluid diet is used mostly when the gastrointestinal tract needs to rest for a few days. It can also be used during the management of an acute diverticulitis attack.

However, in severe cases with significant discomfort and pain, consult your doctor. It may be more appropriate to get admitted to the hospital and receive IV fluids and antibiotics.

Foods and Fluids Allowed on a Clear Fluid Diet

A clear fluid diet includes fluids that are liquid at room temperature. No solid food is allowed. Suitable options include:

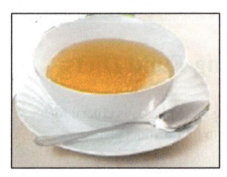

- Tea or Coffee without milk
- Clear juice including green juices (see recipe section for more details).
- Clear jelly
- Clear fizzy drinks such as lemonade
- Electrolyte sports drinks
- Clear popsicles
- Special nutritional supplements such as Ensure Clear, Diabetes Shield, or Boost Breeze (in the USA), and Ensure (in Australia and New Zealand)

Foods and Fluids Not Allowed on a Clear Fluid Diet

The following are not considered clear fluids as they leave residue or food particles behind:
- Milk
- Tomato juice
- Fruit juice with pulp
- Fruit nectar

Example of a Clear Fluid Diet

A clear fluid diet typically lasts two days. It provides only a small amount of energy and is nutrient-deficient, so it should not be used long-term.

Breakfast	Clear tea with two sugars Clear Jelly or Jell-O Ensure Clear (USA) or Ensure (Australia/ NZ)
Morning Tea	Ensure Clear (USA) or Ensure (Australia/ NZ) Ice Block Clear Green Juice
Lunch	Clear Chicken Broth Ensure Clear (USA) or Ensure (Australia/ NZ) Clear Jelly or Jell-O
Afternoon Tea	Ensure Clear (USA) or Ensure (Australia/ NZ)
Dinner	Clear Beef Broth Clear Jelly or Jell-O Ensure Clear (USA) or Ensure (Australia/ NZ)
Supper	Clear tea with two sugars

Note: This is not an endorsement of Ensure products but is used as an example of what is available in the supermarket. There may be other products around that have no residue after consumption.

The graph below (a nutritional analysis of the menu above) shows that the clear fluid diet is incomplete. Thus, it is important not to be on this diet for more than a few days.

RDI Comparison for 60 year old Female (70kg, 1.62m)

- Energy: 67% DEER
- Protein: 81%
- Thiamin
- Riboflavin
- Niacin.Eq: 76%
- Vitamin C: 0%
- Vit.B6: 1%
- Vit.B12: 27%
- Folate-DFE: 8%
- Tot.Vit.A.Eq: 0%
- Magnesium: 21%
- Calcium: 19%
- Phosphorus: 111%
- Iron
- Zinc
- Selenium: 125%
- Iodine
- Molybdenum

Graph: Nutritional Analysis of Clear Fluid Menu

The clear fluid menu given as an example above only provides 5003kJ Energy and 42.6g of protein.

Free Fluid Diet

Transition to a Free Fluid Diet

After a couple of days on a clear fluid diet, you should progress to a free fluid diet. You can manage this at home, but consult your GP if you experience a fever or feel unwell.

What is a Free Fluid Diet?

A free fluid diet includes all the items allowed in a clear fluid diet, plus additional items like milk and milk products. This traditionally includes:

Clear broth or Green juices	Milkshakes
Custard	Nurtitional Suppliments: Ensure Clear or Plus
Jelly or Jello	Plain ice cream
Milk	Plain yogurt

Example of a Free Fluid Diet (standard population)

Breakfast	Tea with Milk Clear Jelly or Jell-O Ensure Plus
Morning Tea	Green Vegetable Juice Plain yogurt
Lunch	Clear Chicken Broth or Clear Green Vegetable Juice Ensure Plus Clear Jelly or Jell-O
Afternoon Tea	Tea with milk Ensure Plus
Dinner	Clear Beef Broth or Clear Green Vegetable Juice Clear Jelly or Jell-O with ice cream Ensure Plus
Supper	Tea with Milk

Note: This is not an endorsement of Ensure products but is used as an example of what is available in supermarkets, e.g. Complan or Vitaplan in Australia and New Zealand.

The green vegetable juice recipes are given in section 2 under recipes.

The graph below (a nutritional analysis of the menu above) shows that the free-fluid diet is not complete. Thus, it is important not to be on this diet for more than a few days.

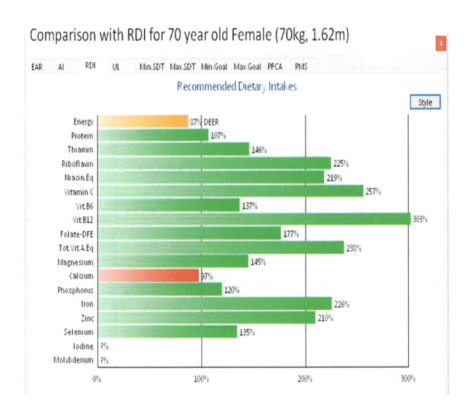

Graph: Nutritional analysis of a free fluid diet

While this diet may provide more protein if you have the right nutritional supplement, it is still insufficient in calories or nutrients for long-term use. Thus, starting on phase 3 is recommended.

Example of a Diabetic Free Fluid Diet

Breakfast	Tea with Milk Diabetic Jelly or Low Sugar Jell-O Glucerna Drink
Morning Tea	Tea with milk Plain yogurt
Lunch	Clear Chicken Broth Diabetic Jelly or Low Sugar Jell-O Glucerna Drink
Afternoon Tea	Tea with milk Glucerna Drink
Dinner	Clear Beef Broth Diabetic Jelly or Low Sugar Jell-O Low Sugar Ice Cream or Sorbet Glucerna Drink
Supper	Tea with Milk

Note: Again, this is not an endorsement of Glucerna as a product but is used as an example of what is available in supermarkets.

You can try some of the green vegetable juices given in the recipe section but check to see that your blood sugar remains within normal range 2 hours after a drink (just to make sure you do not get a hypoglycemic response. I do not think you will but I recommend the side of precaution).

The graph below (a nutritional analysis of the menu above) shows that the free-fluid diet is not complete. Thus, it is important not to be on this diet for more than a few days.

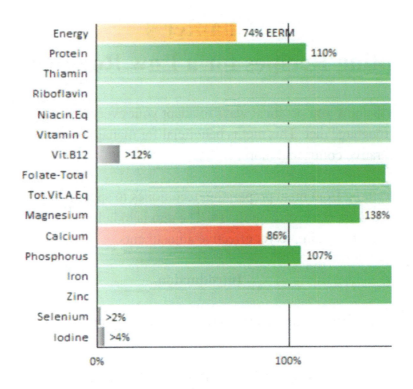

Graph: Nutritional analysis of a diabetic free fluid diet

Summary

This chapter has provided valuable insights into managing diverticulitis through the implementation of fluid diets. By understanding the clear and free-fluid diets, you can give your gastrointestinal tract the rest it needs during an acute attack, allowing for a smoother recovery process.

Remember, these dietary adjustments are essential to managing diverticulitis, but they should be tailored to your individual needs. Always consult your GP for personalized advice and guidance. Clear and free fluid diets are designed to be short-term solutions that provide relief and aid in the healing process.

As you progress through these dietary phases, remember the importance of listening to your body and adjusting as necessary. This knowledge empowers you to take control of your condition and improve your quality of life. Stay proactive, stay informed, and, most importantly, stay healthy.

Thank you for reading this chapter. I hope you find these guidelines helpful and supportive in your journey toward better health and well-being. Take care and continue to prioritize your health as you navigate the challenges of living with diverticulitis.

Chapter 4
Adapting Recipes for a Low Roughage Diet

In this chapter, I will show you practical ways to adapt your everyday foods, making them suitable for a low-roughage diet. This diet is beneficial for managing diverticulitis and helps with conditions like ulcerative colitis and more.

We will cover everything from meal preparation techniques to specific ingredient substitutions that reduce roughage without sacrificing flavor. The aim is to help you enjoy your meals and live life fully while making these simple yet effective adjustments.

Introduction

In acute stage, those suffering from diverticulitis, may benefit from a clear fluid diet with antibiotics for up to two days.

Clear fluid diet includes jelly, clear juice, clear broths, and clear nutritional supplements such as Ensure Clear.

As the inflammation is brought under control, a free fluid diet may be initiated.

After this, a low roughage diet that is low in insoluble fiber or resistant starch is introduced. The aim of a low roughage diet is to keep the fecal bulk to a minimum so that there is not a lot of pressure on the affected area.

A low roughage diet is recommended for up to 21 days after which a transition to high fiber diet is recommended.

What Is A Low Roughage Diet?

Dietary fiber is a group of carbohydrate that cannot be digested by the enzymes that break down carbohydrate. They are found in fruit, vegetables, nuts, lentils, legumes, and grains.

There are three forms of fiber: insoluble fiber (does not dissolve in water), soluble fiber (which dissolves in water) and resistant starch.

Sources of soluble fiber are: rolled oats, peeled apples, carrots, barley.

Sources of insoluble fiber include nuts, whole grain, unbroken grains, fibrous parts of cauliflower, cabbage, broccoli etc.

A diet can be high in soluble fiber but low in insoluble fiber (This diet is called a low roughage diet).

In case of diverticulitis, in the transition phase from fluid diet to high fiber diet, it is recommended a balanced diet low in insoluble fiber (or Low Roughage Diet) is followed for a short period of time (for up to 21 days) after an acute inflammatory episode.

Recent research does not support avoidance of nuts and seeds during well stage. One preventative habit is to chew all food in the mouth till it is smooth. Maximised Nutrition Limited is a bit more cautious and advises that if patient experience shows that symptoms of flare are related to certain foods, then to avoid these foods.

Note: Many of the diverticulitis management diet plans talk about a low residue diet. This is not the approach I take.

A low roughage diet is different from a low residue diet. A low residue diet means that there is minimum residue or bulk left after fiber is digested. A low roughage diet however, takes out the gritty, undigestible fibers from the diet (the parts that could irritate an inflamed gut surface) but allows bulk to be formed after digestion is completed.

We still want fiber so that we can feed the gut microbiome but we want them to be high in soluble fiber (leaving minimum residue in the gut).

Adapting Common Food To A Low Roughage Option

We can use certain foods that have insoluble fiber by adapting how we prepare them for cooking and consumption. Below are some examples.

Flavoring with Low Roughage

Garlic and Onion
Garlic and Onion add deliciousness to our cooking. Normal garlic is high in roughage, but you can pound it and filter out the rough parts using a sieve. You can make your own flavored oils using onion and garlic.

Step 1: Pound or fine-chop onion or garlic.
Step 2: Add to a cup of oil in a pot.
Step 3: Simmer to extract oil.
Step 4: Allow to cool
Step 5: Use a sieve and extract flavored oil. Discard tough fibers.
Step 5: Pour into a sterilized, airtight glass bottle and use for cooking as needed.

Italian Herb Infused Oil

For this you need:

1 cup of Olive Oil
6 leaves of basil
2 sprigs (around 1 tablespoon) of fresh thyme
2 sprigs (around 1 tablespoon) of fresh rosemary
2 sprigs (around 1 tablespoon) of fresh oregano
(if you do not have fresh herbs, pound 1 tsp each of the above using mortar and pestle with some oil).

Add the above to the cup of olive oil. And place in an air-tight bottle. Use within 2 to 3 days. I like to leave this for a day to allow the herbs to infuse into the oil. When using the herb infused oil, just use the oil, sieving off the herb part of it.

This is great to use in the homemade creme of tomato soup.

Indian Spice Infused Oil

For this recipe, you will need the following:

3 tablespoons whole coriander seeds
2-3 whole cloves
2 tablespoons whole cumin seeds
1 two-inch piece cinnamon stick (break into smaller bits)
10 whole green cardamom pods
5 bay leaves or curry leaves (curry leaves are different from bay leaves).
1 tablespoon ground turmeric
2 cup olive oil

1. In a heavy bottomed pan, add the cumin seeds, the coriander seeds, cinnamon sticks, whole cloves.
2. Lightly toast for two minutes. Remove from heat.
3. Place in a grinder or a pastel and motor and grind to fine powder.
4. Add these with turmeric and bay leaves in oil and put in an air tight bottle. It can keep for two weeks.
5. Before using it for cooking, use a fine sieve and remove any debris or residue.

Vegetable Preparation

Brocolli

Cut the florets to reduce fiber content. Boil to soften.

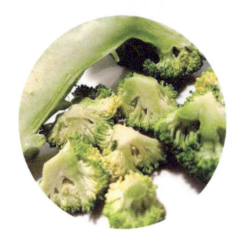

Cauliflower

You can make a puree by boiling or steaming, then blending smooth.

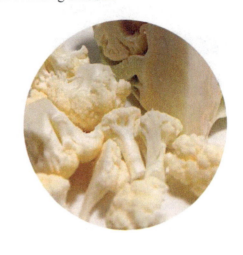

Zucchini and Cucumber

Peel the skin off and remove the seeds to make them low roughage. Eat only the white flesh.

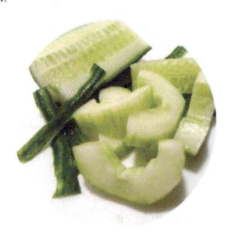

Pumpkin

Remove the skin. Boil, steam, or microwave instead of roasting to keep the fiber soft. If roasting, cook until done but not caramelized.

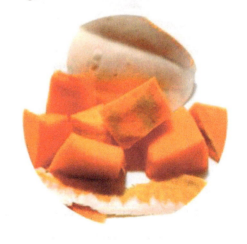

Silverbeet (Swiss Chard) 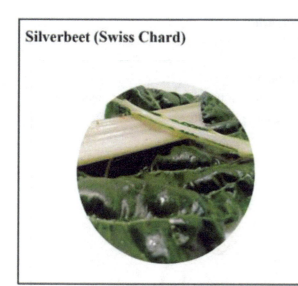	Use the leaves and cut off the white stems to reduce roughage content.

Fruit Preparation

Apple or Pear 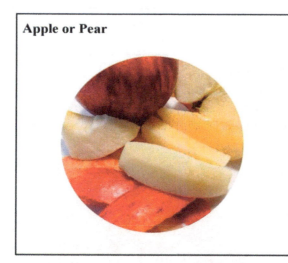	Remove the skin and seeds. Stew the apple for easier digestion and bottle it in sterilized containers for food safety.

Snack Options

Fruit Rolls or Plain Muffins

Choose soft fruit rolls without seeds. Plain fine flour muffins such as chocolate muffins, vanilla muffins, Madeira cake or sponge cakes are okay.

Herbs and Seasonings

Onion, Garlic, and Parsley

Use a pastel and mortar to pound them to extract essential oils and flavors, making them easier to digest. Then, use a sieve to remove the extract and discard the fiber.

Cumin

Ground cumin is preferable to whole seeds for a low roughage diet.

Soups

Cream Soups	Make your soups or choose cream soups from the supermarket.
	Use a sieve to remove any roughness before consuming.

Table: Suitable Food Types and Foods Types to Avoid When On A Low Roughage Diet

Category	Suitable Types	Types to Avoid
Bread	White Bread or toast (Oatilicious) Fine Wholemeal Bread High fiber White Bread, English Muffins	Breads with unbroken seeds, whole grains, nuts, kibble wheat Burned or crusty toast
Cereals	Fine Rolled Oats Cornflakes or Rice Bubbles White Rice, Pasta, Sago, Tapioca Cornflour, White Flour	Bran, Muesli, All Bran, Wholemeal Flour, Wholemeal or Whole Grain Pasta, Brown Rice, Wheat Germ Caution with Doughy Foods such as Scones, Very Fresh Bread
Cakes / Biscuits	Plain Sweet Biscuits Ginger Nuts, Shortbread, Rice Cakes, Rice Wafers, Plain Sponge Cakes, Madeira Cake	Wholemeal or bran biscuits, cakes or biscuits with dried fruit, nuts, coconut
Desserts	Jello, Plain desserts, milk puddings yogurt, plain ice cream	Any containing seeds, skins, coconuts, nuts, dried fruit
Fruit	Fruit without skin or seeds such as melon, pawpaw, banana, apples, pears, peaches	Fruit with pips, skin or seeds such as Kiwifruit, strawberries, cranberry, citrus pith and membrane, dried fruit such as figs, sultanas, raisins, currents
Vegetables	Soft vegetables without tough fibers or skins e.g. - Skinless potato, Skinless kumara - Skinless and seedless pumpkin - Skinless beetroot - Soft leaves of Swiss Chard (no stems) - Peeled carrots - Cauliflower tips - Broccoli tips	Corn, baked beans, peas, seeds, skins, pips or course stalks, mushroom, cabbage family, onion, garlic, tomato, beans, broad beans Roasted Vegetables, Fried Chips
Nuts / Seeds	Smooth peanut butter Nutella Finely ground nuts	Crunchy peanut butter Nuts: whole, chopped Sesame seeds, sunflower, poppy or pumpkin seeds
Beverages	Weak tea or coffee. Infused Fruit Flavored Tea. Clear Fruit Juice or Vegetable Juice or Cordial	Fruit Drinks with Pulp
Dairy	All varieties of milk Plain yogurt or custard Plain or flavored ice-cream Cheese	Any containing died fruit, nuts or coconut Shakes etc that have chunky fruit or vegetable pieces Cheeses with nuts or seeds, fruit yogurt with seeds, skins
Fat	All plain spreads or fat such as butter, margarine, cream, oil, plain salad dressing	Rich mayonnaise, rich pastry, batter, fried foods
Meat, Fish, Poultry, Eggs, Nuts, Legumes	Tender meat, fish, poultry, lean bacon or ham. Meat or fish paste, smooth spreads, poached eggs	Tough grisly meats, fried or highly seasoned or herbed meat or meat products e.g. sausages, prepared dried meats such as jerky, fried eggs
Others	Plain gravy Lollies, sugar, honey, plain ice cream toppings	Pop corn

Chapter 5
Introduction to the 21-Day Low Roughage Menu

In this chapter, I will explain how I developed this menu and how you can effectively manage your diverticular disease. We will cover everything from portion sizes tailored to different countries and age groups to specific dietary needs for those with diabetes. Remember, this menu is designed to help you enjoy your meals while managing your condition, ensuring you get the proper nutrients without compromising taste or enjoyment. Let us dive in and explore how these simple adaptations can make a big difference in your daily diet.

For recipes to support all your phases, please refer to section three.

What is the 21-Day Low Roughage Menu?

This section outlines the 21-day low roughage menu for people with diverticular disease. The menu is created for a standard, healthy population and has also adapted for those with diabetes.

Suitability of the Menu

If you have multiple health problems, this menu may not be suitable. In this case, please consult with your health professional. However, it is primarily designed for individuals with diverticular disease. The menu provides information on portion sizes guideline for those living in the United States of America, Australia, and New Zealand by gender and age categories.

Age Categories and Nutritional Requirements

The menu is divided into the following age categories:

- 40 to 50
- 50 to 60
- 60 to 70
- 70 to 80
- 80+

These categories exist because nutritional requirements vary with age. For example, a person over 65 will have higher protein needs than someone in a lower age category.

Country-Specific Considerations

Different countries have different food sources, such as variations in bread ingredients and meat cuts. These differences affect the protein amounts in the meat. The average heights and weights of the population for different countries also differ by age categories. For example, an average 40-year-old to 49-year-old USA female weighs 67kg and has a height 1.62m. An average 40 year to 49-year-old Australian female weighs 71kg and has a height 1.62m. On the other hand, an average New Zealand female weighs 68kg and has a height 1.65m.

Therefore, the menu is analyzed to meet the daily nutritional requirements for the three countries (Australia, New Zealand, and USA) by age and gender (male and female) category. Note though, the nutrition education information and recipes and menus can be used by other countries. The Author only had the analysis program for the three above named countries.

Nutrient Analysis

The data revealed that following the menu using the specified portion sizes will meet the nutritional requirements for most nutrients. However, some subgroups may still lack certain nutrients, which will be discussed in a later section on nutritional supplementation.

Nutritional Differences by Age and Gender

The menus are analyzed to ensure compliance with the recommended daily intake of particular nutrients. For example, following the diet for a female diabetic aged 40 to 50 may result in lower vitamin C intake compared to other age groups. Another example is where a 40-year-old to 50-year-old male needs more calories than a female of the same age, just because of their physical makeup.

Nutritional Supplementation

In a later section, we will discuss the use of multivitamins or other supplements to address potential nutrient deficiencies identified in the analysis. I hope this introduction to the 21-day low roughage menu has been enlightening and helpful. Understanding how to adapt your meals to meet your dietary needs allows you to manage your diverticular disease more effectively while still enjoying delicious and nutritious food.

Go to section 4 for country specific, age specific, gender specific daily meal portion guidelines for the 21 days.

Comments on the Diabetes Menu

Blood sugar levels can increase during flare-up. Thus, the Diabetes menu has been designed to help those with diabetes balance their protein and carbohydrate during the day to regulate the blood sugar level.

Keep a record of your blood sugar reading: half an hour before a meal and 2 hours after a meal if possible and adjust your insulin or medications as needed.

Can You Have Biscuits, Cakes, Muffins etc. As Snacks?

You can have plain biscuits, plain muffins, scones etc. but the way I designed this menu is to ensure that you are meeting your recommended daily allowance/intake of all the nutrients your body needs. This is important to ensure that your body has the nutrients it needs to fight infection and related inflammatory response.

Also note, that with use of antibiotics, your existing gut microbiome will be changed. Feeding refined sugar products potentially can lead to the pathogenic microbiome growing in greater numbers than the beneficial microbiome. By not feeding refined sugar products and increasing intake of prebiotics (found in fruit and vegetables, like the use of green smoothies), you can help the beneficial microbiome to establish well in the gut ecosystem.

Remember there are some good recipe books on the internet on this topic. The difference between this one and the others are that this one is very holistic in its approach and aims to provide country, gender, age specific guidelines to ensure that you meet all your nutritional requirements during each phase of dietary management.

The menu in this book is designed with your health and satisfaction in mind, tailored to various age groups and specific dietary requirements, including those with diabetes. As you implement these changes, always consult your healthcare provider to ensure they suit your needs. Thank you for taking the time to explore these resources, and I hope they contribute positively to your health journey. Take care and enjoy your meals!

Chapter 6
Understanding and Managing Symptomatic Uncomplicated Diverticular Disease (SUDD)

In this chapter, I want to discuss a subclass of diverticular disease that is often overlooked: symptomatic uncomplicated diverticular disease (SUDD). In the first few chapters, we covered a wide range of diverticular conditions, including symptomatic and asymptomatic cases and both complicated and uncomplicated diverticulitis.

Let us now focus on SUDD and its role in chronic inflammation syndrome.

SUDD is a persistent yet often misunderstood condition. Many patients experience ongoing discomfort, such as diarrhea, bloating, irregular bowel movements, gas, and pain, which are frequently misdiagnosed as irritable bowel syndrome (IBS).

However, these symptoms can persist even in the absence of visible inflammation.

Recognizing and correctly diagnosing SUDD is crucial for effective management and improving patient quality of life. This chapter will delve into the causes, current research, and practical treatment options, including dietary adjustments, to help you better understand and manage SUDD.

What is SUDD?

Symptomatic uncomplicated diverticular disease (SUDD) is characterized by persistent abdominal symptoms attributed to diverticula without obvious colitis or diverticulitis. Essentially, there is no visible inflammation, but symptoms such as diarrhea, bloating, irregular bowel movements, gas, and ongoing pain persist even after antibiotic treatment. Often, these symptoms are misdiagnosed as irritable bowel syndrome (IBS), but they indicate SUDD.

Understanding Chronic Inflammation Syndrome

To understand SUDD, it is essential to understand the structure of your bowel and how it functions.

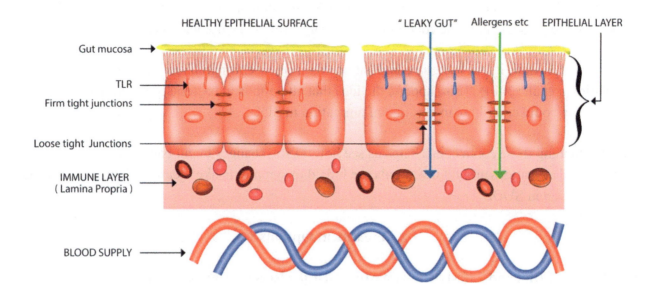

Your colon has a thin layer of epithelial cells that separates the intestinal contents from the rest of your body. This epithelial layer is protected by a mucus layer, which acts as a barrier against acids, chemicals, and food particles. There are toll-like receptors (TLR) in the epithelial layer. These receptors act like security gate that get stimulated by what is in the gut environment. Between the cells are firm tight junctions, like tight connectors that keep the cells tightly fitted with one another. Underneath the epithelial layer is the lamina propria, a loose connective tissue that allows immune cells and inflammation markers to float through, preventing harmful substances from invading your body. Under this, is the blood supply.

Role of Toll-Like Receptors In SUDD

Toll-like receptors (TLRs) are like the body's security guards, helping to spot trouble in the gut. In symptomatic uncomplicated diverticular disease (SUDD), these guards become extra sensitive, especially around the diverticula.

Now, imagine these diverticula as little pockets in the colon wall. In SUDD, the tissue around these pockets changes, becoming more prone to inflammation. TLRs in these areas become more active, ready to react to any potential threats. When the TLR start getting more active, the tight junctions that hold the cells closely together become looser, thus allowing particles, allergens, irritants etc. to travel freely from the gut into the body itself.

As a result of these changes, the types of bacteria living around these diverticula can also change. Normally, our gut has a diverse community of bacteria, but in SUDD, this balance can shift. Some types of bacteria may thrive more in these altered areas, potentially worsening inflammation and symptoms like bloating, pain, and chronic inflammation.

For example, Barbara et al. (2010) found that TLRs are more active in people with SUDD compared to those without the condition, suggesting a role in symptom development.

Moreover, changes in gut bacteria composition can influence inflammation, as shown in a study by Colman et al. (2014). This supports the idea that alterations in bacteria types around diverticula could contribute to chronic inflammation in SUDD.

Understanding these connections helps us see how TLRs, changes in gut bacteria, and anatomical alterations around diverticula are linked to symptoms like bloating, pain, and chronic inflammation in SUDD.

Treatment Options

Influence of Diet and Lifestyle Factors In Toll-Like Receptor Function in SUDD

Now, here's how diet and lifestyle can influence TLR functions in SUDD:

Dietary Fiber

Eating a diet low in fiber is a common risk factor for developing diverticular disease. Fiber helps keep the digestive system healthy and can influence the types of bacteria living in the gut. Studies suggest that a low-fiber diet can alter the gut microbiota composition, potentially affecting TLR activation and inflammation (Raskov et al., 2019).

Obesity

Being overweight or obese is also associated with an increased risk of diverticular disease. Obesity can lead to chronic low-grade inflammation in the body, which may affect TLR functions and contribute to inflammation in SUDD (Caviglia et al., 2017).

Physical Activity

Regular physical activity has been linked to a reduced risk of diverticular disease. Exercise can help maintain a healthy weight and reduce inflammation in the body, which may influence TLR functions (Humes et al., 2019).

Smoking

Smoking is another risk factor for diverticular disease. It can disrupt the balance of bacteria in the gut and promote inflammation, potentially affecting TLR activation (Tursi, 2016).

Making dietary and lifestyle changes, such as increasing fiber intake, maintaining a healthy weight, being physically active, and avoiding smoking, can help modulate TLR functions and reduce inflammation in SUDD.

Studies have found that antibiotics, such as rifaximin, can reduce TLR4 activity, helping to control chronic inflammation. Combining antibiotics with probiotics, which introduce healthy bacteria into the gut, can further improve treatment outcomes. Probiotics, especially those containing gram-positive bacteria, help open the right gates for beneficial substances and close them to harmful ones.

Role of Antibiotics and Probiotics

Antibiotics are medications that fight bacterial infections. In SUDD, antibiotics like Rifaximin can help reduce symptoms by targeting harmful bacteria in the gut. By reducing the number of harmful bacteria, antibiotics may also decrease the activation of Toll-like receptors (TLRs), which are like the body's alarm system for detecting invaders. This can help reduce inflammation and symptoms in SUDD (Tursi et al., 2016).

Probiotics are beneficial bacteria that can help restore balance in the gut microbiota. Certain strains of probiotics, such as Bifidobacterium and Lactobacillus species, have been studied for their effects on TLR functions in SUDD. These probiotics may help regulate TLR activation and reduce inflammation in the gut, leading to improved symptoms (Losurdo et al., 2015).

Importance of Prebiotics

Prebiotics are non-digestible fibers that servings of as food for beneficial bacteria in the gut. By promoting the growth of beneficial bacteria, prebiotics can indirectly influence TLR functions. Prebiotics may help modulate TLR activation and reduce inflammation in conditions like SUDD (Barbara et al., 2019).

Incorporating prebiotic fibers into your diet can also support healthy gut bacteria.

Prebiotics are found in a variety of fruits and vegetables, and consuming a diverse range of these foods can promote the growth of beneficial bacteria. Prebiotics like those found in apples, onions, broccoli, and cauliflower can help maintain gut health.

So, antibiotics like Rifaximin can directly target harmful bacteria and reduce TLR activation, while probiotics and prebiotics can promote a healthier balance of gut bacteria, indirectly influencing TLR functions and inflammation in SUDD.

Practical Application

Thus, even as you use the 21-day Low Roughage Menu for Phase 2 management of diverticulitis, it may be helpful to incorporate a probiotic and prebiotic fibers in your diet, especially if you have symptoms of bloating, pain, and nausea. Remember to choose a probiotic blend that has a range of strains including Bifidobacterium and Lactobacillus species in it.

References

Barbara, G., et al. (2010). Toll-like receptor 2 and 4 expression in the intestinal mucosa of patients with symptomatic uncomplicated diverticular disease. BMC Gastroenterology, 10, 10. doi:10.1186/1471-230x-10-10

Barbara, G., Scaioli, E., Barbaro, M. R., Biagi, E., Laghi, L., Cremon, C., Corinaldesi, R. (2019). Gut microbiota, metabolome, and immune signatures in patients with uncomplicated diverticular disease. Gut, 68(6), 1083–1093. doi:10.1136/gutjnl-2018-316304

Caviglia, G. P., Rosso, C., Ribaldone, D. G., Dughera, F., Fagoonee, S., & Pellicano, R. (2017). The Role of Diet in the Pathogenesis of Colonic Diverticular Disease: Is There an Evidence-Based Relationship? Nutrients, 9(8), 805. doi:10.3390/nu9080805

Colman, R. J., et al. (2014). The commensal microbiota influences the susceptibility to colitis and colitis-associated colorectal cancer in IL-10-/- mice. Inflammatory Bowel Diseases, 20(12), 2319–2328. doi:10.1097/mib.0000000000000247

Humes, D. J., Fleming, K. M., Spiller, R. C., & West, J. (2019). Concurrent drug use and the risk of perforated colonic diverticular disease: a population-based case-control study. Gut, 68(6), 1014–1020. doi:10.1136/gutjnl-2018-317829

Losurdo, G., Principi, M., Girardi, B., & Fiore, M. G. (2015). Probiotic monotherapy and Helicobacter pylori eradication: A systematic review with pooled-data analysis. World Journal of Gastroenterology, 21(10), 2512–2520. doi:10.3748/wjg.v21.i10.2512

Raskov, H., Burcharth, J., Pommergaard, H. C., & Rosenberg, J. (2019). Irritable bowel syndrome, the microbiota, and the gut-brain axis. Gut Microbes, 10(3), 224–236. doi:10.1080/19490976.2018.1515041

Tursi, A. (2016). Smoking in diverticular disease: A systematic review of the evidence. Colorectal Disease, 18(6), 528–539. doi:10.1111/codi.13307

Tursi, A., Brandimarte, G., Giorgetti, G. M., & Elisei, W. (2016). Assessment and grading of mucosal inflammation in colonic diverticular disease. Journal of Clinical Gastroenterology, 50(Suppl 1), S18–S22. doi:10.1097/mcg.0000000000000614

Chapter 7
Development of SIBO/IMO in Diverticular Disease

Small intestinal bacterial overgrowth (SIBO) and intestinal methanogen overgrowth (IMO) are conditions where there is an excess of bacteria, often from the colon, in the small intestine. This can happen in diverticular disease, where small pouches (diverticula) form in the colon wall.

How SIBO/IMO Can Develop In Diverticulitis

Diverticula Formation

Diverticula are like little pockets that form in the colon wall. They can trap food and bacteria, creating a breeding ground for bacterial overgrowth.

Altered Motility

In diverticular disease, the movement of the intestines can change. This can slow down the passage of food and bacteria, allowing them to accumulate and overgrow.

Stagnation of Contents

Food and bacteria can get stuck in the diverticula, creating stagnant areas where bacteria can thrive.

Bacterial Overgrowth

With the excess of bacteria in the colon, some can migrate backward into the small intestine or accumulate in the diverticula.

Fermentation

Once in the small intestine or diverticula, these bacteria ferment undigested carbohydrates, producing gases like hydrogen and methane. Methane-producing bacteria can also overgrow in the small intestine, leading to IMO.

Symptoms: SIBO/IMO can cause symptoms like bloating, abdominal discomfort, and changes in bowel habits, which are common in diverticular disease.

SIBO/IMO Treatment Options

Antibiotics

Antibiotics like Rifaximin can help by reducing the number of bacteria in the small intestine. This can improve symptoms and reduce bacterial fermentation.

Probiotics

Probiotics are beneficial bacteria that can help restore balance in the gut. Certain strains, like Bifidobacterium and Lactobacillus, have been studied for their potential to reduce bacterial overgrowth and improve symptoms in SIBO/IMO.

Dietary Modifications

Dietary changes can help manage SIBO/IMO. Avoiding fermentable carbohydrates that feed bacteria, known as the low FODMAP diet, may help reduce symptoms. Increasing fiber intake can also help by promoting regular bowel movements and preventing bacterial overgrowth.

Prokinetics

Prokinetic agents can improve intestinal motility, helping to move food and bacteria through the digestive tract more efficiently. This can reduce the risk of bacterial overgrowth and alleviate symptoms. Ginger is an example of a natural prokinetic.

If you have tried this four-stage dietary management plan for diverticulitis, and you still have symptoms of bloating, pain, etc., it may be that you have SIBO/IMO. Thus, a hydrogen methane breath test is recommended to see if you have SIBO/IMO. See articles on Hydrogen Methane Breath Tests on the website of Maximised Nutrition (maximisednutrition.com).

By addressing the underlying bacterial overgrowth and motility issues, these treatment options can help manage SIBO/IMO and improve symptoms in diverticular disease.

References

Losurdo, G., et al. (2015). Probiotic monotherapy and Helicobacter pylori eradication: A systematic review with pooled-data analysis. World Journal of Gastroenterology, 21(10), 2512–2520. doi:10.3748/wjg.v21.i10.2512

Pimentel, M., et al. (2006). Treatment of irritable bowel syndrome with rifaximin in clinical practice: A single center experience. Alimentary Pharmacology & Therapeutics, 24(4), 675–684. doi:10.1111/j.1365-2036.2006.03096.x

Rezaie, A., et al. (2017). Hydrogen and methane-based breath testing in gastrointestinal disorders: The North American consensus. The American Journal of Gastroenterology, 112(5), 775–784. doi:10.1038/ajg.2017.46

Chapter 8
Preventing Diverticulitis: Strategies and Tips

In this chapter, I will discuss how to prevent diverticula from developing and what to do after a diverticulitis episode to prevent recurrence. Diverticulitis is a condition that can significantly impact your quality of life, but with the right knowledge and practices, you can reduce your risk and manage the condition effectively.

Understanding the factors that predispose individuals to diverticulitis is crucial for effective prevention. We will explore essential lifestyle and dietary changes that can help you maintain a healthy digestive system and avoid diverticular disease. Incorporating these strategies into your daily routine can improve your overall health and well-being while minimizing the risk of diverticulitis. Let us dive into these preventative measures and tips to help you lead a healthier, more comfortable life.

Factors that Contribute to the Development of Diverticula

Several factors can increase the risk of developing diverticula:

Obesity and Overweight

Maintaining a healthy weight is essential. Aim for a BMI of 20 to 25 or 20 to 28 if you are older or have a larger build. Keeping a lean waist-to-hip ratio is beneficial. Excess body weight, especially around the abdomen, increases pressure on the colon, which can lead to the formation of diverticula. Regular physical activity and a balanced diet are vital components in achieving and maintaining a healthy weight.

Smoking

Smokers have a higher risk of developing diverticula. Smoking affects overall gut health and can lead to inflammation and weakened intestinal walls. Quitting smoking can significantly reduce your risk of developing diverticular disease and improve your overall health.

High Red Meat Intake

Limit red meat to 2 to 3 times a week. Opt for chicken, fish, and a variety of legumes instead. Diets high in red meat have been associated with increased inflammation and altered gut microbiota, which can contribute to diverticular disease. Incorporating more plant-based proteins and lean meats can help maintain a healthy digestive system.

Certain Drugs

Medications such as aspirin, NSAIDs, corticosteroids, and opiates can predispose individuals to diverticula. These drugs can irritate the intestinal lining and disrupt the balance of gut bacteria. If you need to take these medications, discuss with your healthcare provider about ways to minimize their impact on your gut health.

Preventative Measures

To reduce the risk of developing diverticula, consider the following preventative measures:

Vigorous Exercise

Engage in activities that make you sweat, such as running, cycling, swimming, or aerobic exercise. Regular vigorous exercise is beneficial for overall health and can help prevent diverticular disease. Exercise helps maintain a healthy weight, reduces inflammation, and promotes regular bowel movements, all of which are important for digestive health.

High-fiber diet

Consume 200 to 300 grams of fruits and vegetables daily, aiming for 9 servings to 11 servings each day. A serving is equivalent to the size of your hand when you are holding an object the size of an orange. A high-fiber diet helps maintain bowel health, prevents constipation, and promotes the growth of beneficial bacteria. Fiber adds bulk to the stool, making it easier to pass and reducing the pressure on the colon walls. Whole grains, nuts, seeds, and legumes are also excellent sources of fiber.

Since the start of diverticulitis may be due to an imbalance of gut microbiome, including green vegetables such as broccoli, spinach, kale, Swiss chard/Silverbeet, Bok choy etc. and as many colors of other fruit and vegetables provide a whole lot of prebiotic fibers that are foods to your gut bacteria. Thus, regular intake of green vegetable smoothies is also recommended. Always try to have one green vegetable with your dinner meals every night.

Vitamin D

Increase your vitamin D levels by spending 10 to 20 minutes in the sun each day, preferably in the morning or evening. Always protect your skin when exposed to the sun. Vitamin D plays a role in immune function and inflammation regulation. You can also get vitamin D from foods like fatty fish, fortified dairy products, and supplements.

Alcohol

The relationship between alcohol consumption and diverticular disease is still under investigation. It is best to consume alcohol in moderation and monitor its effects on your digestive health. Excessive alcohol intake can irritate the digestive tract and alter gut microbiota, increasing the risk of diverticular disease.

Dietary Tips

Avoid Nuts and High-Fiber Foods During Acute Episodes

If you experience an acute diverticulitis episode with bleeding or severe pain, avoid nuts and high-fiber foods to prevent irritation. During these times, a low-roughage diet can help reduce inflammation and allow the colon to heal.

Personalized Diet

Be aware of your symptoms and identify foods that cause discomfort. Some individuals may find that spicy foods or certain nuts exacerbate their symptoms. Keeping a food diary can help you track which foods trigger your symptoms and adjust your diet accordingly.

For most people, with no symptoms, in well stage, a Mediterranean diet option is suitable.

Variety and Balance

Maintain a balanced diet with a variety of foods. Avoid overly restrictive diets to ensure you receive adequate nutrition. Eating a diverse range of fruits, vegetables, grains, and proteins ensures you get all the essential nutrients your body needs for optimal health. The best dietary style to eat for healthy living is the Mediterranean Diet, which is a wholesome, high-fiber diet where protein sources are mainly from chicken, fish, lentils, legumes, chickpeas with some red meat, high in healthy fat, moderate in the amount of carbohydrate and protein.

Additional Preventative Strategies

Hydration

Drink plenty of water throughout the day. Staying hydrated helps your digestive system function smoothly and prevents constipation, which can exacerbate diverticular issues. Aim for at least 8 cups of water a day, more if you are active or live in a hot climate.

Regular Medical Check-Ups

Regular visits to your healthcare provider can help monitor your condition and make necessary adjustments to your diet and lifestyle. Early detection and management of potential issues can prevent complications.

Stress Management

Chronic stress can negatively affect your digestive health. Incorporate stress management techniques such as meditation/prayer, or deep breathing exercises into your daily routine.

Finding healthy ways to manage stress can improve overall well-being and reduce the risk of digestive issues.

Social Engagement
Social engagement and social connectedness are key elements of positive health insofar as they reduce stress, improve mental well-being, and lower the risk of chronic diseases. Meaningful interactions not only enable individual resilience but also reinforce healthy behaviors, create emotional support networks, and lead to overall better health and longevity, enriching them with a feeling of belonging and purpose.

Regular Exercise
Regular exercise drastically cuts down on stress by prompting the release of endorphins, which are natural mood lifters and help with easing anxiety. It controls cortisol, a stress hormone in the body, in order to avoid chronic stress. Exercise promotes gut health through improvements in gut motility, reduced inflammation, and facilitating the growth of beneficial bacteria that may improve digestion and immunity. Exercise that requires oxygen, such as walking and cycling, was found to have beneficial effects on the gut microbiome through the increase in production of short-chain fatty acids that ensure the health and balance of the gut.

Probiotics & Prebiotics

Consider incorporating probiotics and prebiotics into your diet through supplements or foods like yogurt, kefir, and fermented vegetables. Probiotics can help the existing beneficial bacteria to grow in the gut. Prebiotics (found in apple, chicory, dandelion greens, asparagus, and artichokes) feed the existing microbiome and help them to grow. A healthy gut microbiome supports digestion and can reduce inflammation.

Summary

Implementing these preventative measures and dietary tips can help reduce your risk of developing diverticula and manage diverticulitis effectively.

Be mindful of your body's responses to different foods and adjust your diet accordingly.

If you need personalized advice, especially for Australian and New Zealand clients, consider booking an online consultation for a discounted rate on my website: maximisednutrition.com.

Regular check-ups with your healthcare provider can also help manage your condition effectively.

Take care, stay healthy, and be proactive in managing diverticulitis. Incorporating these strategies into your daily routine can significantly improve your quality of life and reduce the risk of diverticular disease.

SECTION TWO
21 Day Standard and Diabetic Menus and Shopping Lists

Standard Population

Week 1 Menu For Standard Population

Category	Monday	Tuesday	Wednesday	Thursday	Friday	Saturday	Sunday
			**BREAKFAST**				
Cereals		Rice Bubbles (Rice Krispies) OR Porridge with Sugar OR Cornflakes					
Dairy		Low Fat Milk OR Whole Milk OR Plain or Fruit Flavored yogurt					
		Peaches - Stewed	Pears - Stewed	Apples - Stewed	Pears - Stewed	Peaches - Stewed	Apples - Stewed	Peaches - Stewed
		Fruit Juice					
Breads		White Toast OR White Bread OR Whole Meal Bread					
Spreads		Margarine or Butter or Avocado Spread With Honey OR Peanut Butter (Smooth) OR Apricot Jam Nutritional Yeast for Extra B Vitamins					
		Clear Fruit Juice					
		*Morning Tea (choose 1 option)*					
Morning Tea		Plain Crackers & Cheese	Plain Crackers & Cheese	Plain Cracker, Cottage Cheese	Plain Cracker, Cottage Cheese	Plain Crackers and Cream Cheese	Plain Crackers & Cheese	Plain Natural yogurt
		OR Plain Biscuits					
		**LUNCH**					
Soup		Cream of Pumpkin	Crème of Tomato	Crème of Tomato	Cream of Chicken	Crème of Tomato	Cream of Pumpkin	Crème of Tomato
		*Sandwich (made with white or wholemeal bread)*					
Sandwich		Ham	Egg	Beef	Ham	Chicken	CornedSilverside	Cheese
		*Extra*					
Bakery		White Bread OR Rice Wafer OR Wholemeal Bread					
Spreads		Butter or Margarine or Avocado Spread With Peanut Butter (smooth) OR Apricot Jam					
		*Fresh Fruit* *Soft Banana*					
		*Afternoon Tea (choose 1 option)*					
Afternoon Tea		Plain Crackers Cottage Cheese	Plain Crackers & Cream Cheese	Plain yogurt	Plain yogurt	Plain Crackers & Cheese	Plain Crackers and Cream Cheese	Plain Crackers & Cheese
		OR Plain Biscuits or Banana					
		**DINNER**					
		Citrus Salmon, Pea Puree, Mashed Sweet Potato	Beef Burger	Apricot Chicken with Steamed Rice	Creamy Prawn Pasta	Braised Lamb Chop with Rice	Beef Meatball in Tortilla Wrap with Carrot, Cucumber,	Roast Pork, Mashed Potato, Boiled Pumpkin Swiss Chard / Silverbeet
		Salt AND/OR Pepper					
		*Dessert (choose maximum of 2 Options)*					
		Custard or Ice Cream (plain) with Jelly					
		Pears - Stewed	Peaches - Stewed	Pears - Stewed	Peaches - Stewed	Apples - Stewed with Cinnamon	Pears - Stewed	Apples - Stewed with Cinnamon
		*Supper (choose 1 option)*					
Supper		Plain Crackers, Cottage Cheese	Fruit Flavored yogurt	Plain Crackers & Cheese	Plain Crackers & Cheese	Fruit Flavored yogurt	Fruit Flavored yogurt	Plain Crackers & Cream Cheese
		Or Plain Biscuit with A Hot Milky Cocoa Drink					

For Morning Tea, Afternoon Tea, Supper, a hot chocolate option is recommended at times

Week 2 Menu for Standard Population

Category	Monday	Tuesday	Wednesday	Thursday	Friday	Saturday	Sunday
	BREAKFAST						
Cereals	Rice Bubbles (Rice Krispies) OR Porridge with Sugar OR Cornflakes						
Dairy	Low Fat Milk OR Whole Milk OR Plain or Fruit Flavored yogurt						
	Peaches - Stewed	Pears - Stewed	Apples - Stewed	Pears - Stewed	Peaches - Stewed	Apples - Stewed	Peaches - Stewed
	Fruit Juice						
Breads	White Toast OR White Bread OR Whole Meal Bread						
Spreads	Margarine or Butter or Avocado Spread With Honey OR Peanut Butter (Smooth) OR Apricot Jam Nutritional Yeast for Extra B Vitamins						
	Clear Fruit Juice						
	Morning Tea (choose 1 option)						
Morning Tea	Plain Crackers & Cheese	Plain Crackers & Cheese	Plain Cracker, Cottage Cheese	Plain Cracker, Cottage Cheese	Plain Crackers and Cream Cheese	Plain Crackers & Cheese	Plain Natural yogurt
	OR Plain Biscuits						
	LUNCH						
Soup	Cream of Pumpkin	Crème of Tomato	Crème of Tomato	Crème of Chicken	Crème of Tomato	Cream of Pumpkin	Crème of Tomato
	Sandwich (made with white or wholemeal bread)						
Sandwich	Ham	Egg	Beef	Ham	Chicken	CornedSilverside	Cheese
	Extra						
Bakery	White Bread OR Rice Wafer OR Wholemeal Bread						
Spreads	Butter or Margarine or Avocado Spread With Peanut Butter (smooth) OR Apricot Jam						
	Fresh Fruit Soft Banana						
	Afternoon Tea (choose 1 option)						
Afternoon Tea	Plain Crackers Cottage Cheese	Plain Crackers & Cream Cheese	Plain yogurt	Plain yogurt	Plain Crackers & Cheese	Plain Crackers and Cream Cheese	Plain Crackers & Cheese
	OR Plain Biscuits or Banana						
	DINNER						
	Citrus Salmon, Pea Puree, Mashed Sweet Potato	Beef Burger	Apricot Chicken with Steamed Rice	Creamy Prawn Pasta	Braised Lamb Chop with Rice	Beef Meatball in Tortilla Wrap with Carrot, Cucumber,	Roast Pork, Mashed Potato, Boiled Pumpkin Swiss Chard / Silverbeet
	Salt AND/OR Pepper						
	Dessert (choose maximum of 2 Options)						
	Custard or Ice Cream (plain) with Jelly						
	Pears - Stewed	Peaches - Stewed	Pears - Stewed	Peaches - Stewed	Apples - Stewed with Cinnamon	Pears - Stewed	Apples - Stewed with Cinnamon
	Supper (choose 1 option)						
Supper	Plain Crackers, Cottage Cheese	Fruit Flavored yogurt	Plain Crackers & Cheese	Plain Crackers & Cheese	Fruit Flavored yogurt	Fruit Flavored yogurt	Plain Crackers & Cream Cheese
	Or Plain Biscuit with A Hot Milky Cocoa Drink						

For Morning Tea, Afternoon Tea, Supper, a hot chocolate option is recommended at times

Week 3 Menu for Standard Population

Category	Monday	Tuesday	Wednesday	Thursday	Friday	Saturday	Sunday
	BREAKFAST						
Cereals	Rice Bubbles (Rice Krispies) OR Porridge with Sugar OR Cornflakes						
Sugar	Sugar						
	Pears - Stewed	Apples - Stewed	Peaches - Stewed	Apples - Stewed	Peaches - Stewed	Apples - Stewed	Pears - Stewed
	Fruit Juice						
Breads	White Toast OR White Bread OR Whole meal Bread (no seeds or broken grains)						
Spreads	Margarine OR Avocado OR Butter with Honey OR Peanut Butter (Smooth) OR Apricot Jam						
	Nutritional Yeast for Extra Vitamin Bs						
	Morning Tea (choose 1 option)						
Morning Tea	Plain Crackers & Cheese	Plain Crackers & Cheese	Plain Crackers, Cottage Cheese	Plain Crackers, Cottage Cheese	Plain Crackers & Cream Cheese	Plain Crackers & Cheese	Plain Natural yogurt
	OR Plain Biscuits						
	LUNCH						
Soup	Cream of Pumpkin	Crème of Tomato	Cream of Pumpkin	Cream of Chicken	Crème of Tomato	Cream of Pumpkin	Cream of Chicken
	Sandwich (made with white or wholemeal bread)						
Sandwich	Cheese	Tuna	Ham	Corned Beef Silverside	Cheese	Ham	Cheese
	Extra						
Bakery	White Bread OR Rice Wafer OR Wholemeal bread						
Spreads	Margarine OR Avocado OR Butter with Honey OR Peanut Butter (Smooth) OR Apricot Jam						
	Fresh Fruit (soft banana)						
	Afternoon Tea (choose 1 option)						
	Plain yogurt	Plain Crackers, Cream Cheese	Plain yogurt	Plain Crackers Cheese	Plain yogurt	Plain Crackers Cottage Cheese	Plain Crackers & Cream Cheese
	OR Plain Biscuits						
	DINNER						
	Beef Curry with Rice and Spinach	Marinated Pork in Pita Bread	Chicken Chow Mein	Beef Casserole with Steamed Rice	Baked Fish in Coconut Cream with Mashed Potato, Spinach, Carrot	Silverbeet (Swiss Chard) Lamb Lasagna	Chicken Meatballs with Rice, Broccoli, Cauliflower & Parsley Sauce
Condiments	Salt AND/OR Pepper						
Dessert	*Dessert*						
	Custard OR Plain Ice Cream With Jelly						
	Peaches - Stewed	Pears - Stewed	Apples - Stewed with Cinnamon	Peaches - Stewed	Pears - Stewed	Peaches - Stewed	Apples - Stewed with Cinnamon
	Supper (choose 1 option)						
Supper	Plain Crackers & Cheese	Plain yogurt	Plain Crackers & Cheese	Plain yogurt	Plain Crackers & Cheese	Plain yogurt	Plain Crackers & Cheese
	OR Plain Biscuit with Hot Milky Cocoa Drink						

For Morning Tea, Afternoon Tea, Supper, a hot chocolate option is recommended at times

Diabetic Population

Week 1 Menu for Diabetic Population

Category	Monday	Tuesday	Wednesday	Thursday	Friday	Saturday	Sunday
	BREAKFAST						
Cereals	Rice Bubbles (Rice Krispies) OR Porridge with Artificial Sweetener OR Cornflakes						
Dairy	Low Fat Milk OR Whole Milk OR Plain yogurt						
	Peaches – Stewed (drained)	Pears – Stewed (drained)	Apples – Stewed (drained)	Pears – Stewed (drained)	Peaches – Stewed (drained)	Apples – Stewed (drained)	Peaches – Stewed (drained)
	Cordial – sugar free						
Breads	White Toast OR White Bread OR Whole Meal Bread						
Spreads	Margarine OR Butter OR Avocado Spread with Peanut Butter (smooth) OR Diabetic Jam						
	Nutritional Yeast for Extra Vitamin Bs						
	Morning Tea (choose 1 option)						
Morning Tea	Plain Crackers & Cheese	Plain Crackers & Cheese	Plain crackers, cottage cheese	Plain Crackers, Cottage Cheese	Plain Crackers & Cream Cheese	Plain Crackers & Cheese	Plain Crackers, Tuna
	OR Plain Biscuits or digestive with glass of milk						
LUNCH	LUNCH						
Soup	Cream of Pumpkin	Crème of Tomato	Crème of Tomato	Cream of Chicken	Crème of Tomato	Cream of Pumpkin	Crème of Tomato
	Sandwich (made with white or whowhole meal bread)						
Sandwich	Ham	Egg	Beef	Ham	Chicken	Corned Silverside	Cheese
	Extra						
Bakery	White Bread OR Wholemeal Bread OR Rice Wafer						
Spreads	Margarine OR Avocado OR Butter with Peanut Butter (smooth) OR Diabetic Jam						
Fresh Fruit	Allowed Fruit						
	Afternoon Tea (choose 1 option)						
Afternoon Tea	Plain Crackers Cottage Cheese	Plain Crackers & Cream Cheese	Plain yogurt	Plain yogurt	Plain Crackers, & Cheese	Plain Crackers and Cream Cheese	Plain Crackers, & Cheese
	OR Plain Biscuits with glass of milk						
DINNER	DINNER						
	Citrus Salmon with Pea Puree with Mashed Sweet Potato /Kumara	Beef Burger	Apricot Chicken with Steamed Rice	Creamy Prawn Pasta	Braised Lamb Chop with Rice	Beef Meatball in Tortilla Wrap with Cucumber, Carrot	Roast Pork, Mashed Potato, Pumpkin Swiss Chard / Silverbeet
Condiments	Salt AND/OR Pepper						
Dessert	*Dessert (choose maximum of 2 Options)*						
	Custard (sugar free) with Diabetic Jelly						
	Pears – Stewed (drained)	Peaches – Stewed (drained)	Pears – Stewed (drained)	Peaches – Stewed (drained)	Apples - Stewed with Cinnamon (drained)	Pears – Stewed (drained)	Apples - Stewed with Cinnamon (drained)
Supper	Supper						
Supper	Plain Crackers, Cottage Cheese	Plain Crackers, Tuna	Plain Crackers & Cream Cheese	Plain Crackers, Tuna	Plain Crackers, Tuna	Plain Crackers & Cream Cheese	Plain Crackers, Tuna
	With a glass of milk						

If needed for blood sugar control over night, can have a protein sandwich made with white bread for supper.

Week 2 Menu for Diabetic Population

Category	Monday	Tuesday	Wednesday	Thursday	Friday	Saturday	Sunday
			BREAKFAST				
Cereals	Rice Bubbles (Rice Krispies) OR Porridge with Artificial Sweetener OR Cornflakes						
Dairy	Low Fat Milk OR Whole Milk OR Plain yogurt						
	Pears – Stewed (drained)	Apples – Stewed (drained)	Peaches – Stewed (drained)	Apples – Stewed (drained)	Peaches – Stewed (drained)	Apples – Stewed (drained)	Pears – Stewed (drained)
	Cordial – sugar free						
Breads	White Toast OR White Bread OR WHOLEMEAL BREAD (no seeds or broken grains)						
Spreads	Margarine OR Butter OR Avocado Spread with Peanut Butter (smooth) OR Diabetic Jam						
	Morning Tea (choose 1 option)						
	Plain Crackers, & Cheese	Plain Crackers, Cheese	Plain Crackers, Cottage Cheese	Plain Crackers, Cottage Cheese	Plain Crackers & Cream Cheese	Plain Crackers & Cheese	Plain Natural yogurt
	OR Plain or Digestive Biscuits with Glass of Milk						
	LUNCH						
Soup	Cream of Pumpkin	Crème of Tomato	Cream of Pumpkin	Cream of Chicken	Crème of Tomato	Cream of Pumpkin	Cream of Chicken
	Sandwich (made with white or wholemeal bread)						
Sandwich	Cheese	Tuna	Ham	Salmon	Cheese	Ham	Cheese
	Extra						
Bakery	White Bread OR Wholemeal Bread OR Rice Wafer						
Spreads	Plant Based Spread OR Avocado OR Butter with Peanut Butter (smooth) OR Diabetic Jam						
Fresh Fruit	Allowed Fruit						
	Afternoon Tea (choose 1 option)						
	Plain yogurt	Plain Crackers, Cream Cheese	Plain yogurt	Plain Crackers, Cheese	Plain yogurt	Plain Crackers Cottage Cheese	Plain Crackers & Cream Cheese
	OR Plain OR Digestive Biscuits with Milk						
	DINNER						
	Scotch Fillet, Mashed Potato, Steamed Pumpkin & Broccoli	Bacon Egg Potato Top Pie	Moroccan Lamb Shank, Sweet Potato (Kumara), Cucumber, Carrot	Pan Fried Fish with Lemon Slice, Mashed Potato, Cauliflower, Broccoli	Chicken in Basil Sauce	Spaghetti Bolognaise with Broccoli	Corned Silverside, Mashed Potato, Carrot, Swiss Chard (Silverbeet)
Condiments	Salt AND/OR Pepper						
Dessert	**Dessert**						
	Custard – Sugar Free with Diabetic Jelly						
	Peaches – Stewed (drained)	Pears – Stewed (drained)	Apples - Stewed with Cinnamon (drained)	Peaches - Stewed (drained)	Pears – Stewed (drained)	Peaches – Stewed (drained)	Apples - Stewed with Cinnamon (drained)
Supper	**Supper**						
Supper	Plain Crackers & Cream Cheese	Plain Crackers, Tuna	Plain Crackers & Cream Cheese	Plain Crackers, Tuna	Plain Crackers, Tuna	Plain Crackers, Cottage Cheese	Plain Crackers, Tuna
	with a glass of milk						

If needed for blood sugar control over night, can have a protein sandwich made with white bread for supper.

Week 3 Menu for Diabetic Population

Category	Monday	Tuesday	Wednesday	Thursday	Friday	Saturday	Sunday
	BREAKFAST						
Cereals	Rice Bubbles (Rice Krispies) OR Porridge with Artificial Sweetener OR Cornflakes						
Dairy	Low Fat Milk OR Whole Milk OR Plain yogurt						
	Peaches – Stewed (drained)	Pears – Stewed (drained)	Apples – Stewed (drained)	Pears – Stewed (drained)	Peaches - Stewed (drained)	Apples – Stewed (drained)	Peaches – Stewed (drained)
	Cordial – sugar free						
Breads	White Toast OR White Bread OR Wholemeal Bread						
Spreads	Margarine OR Butter with Peanut Butter (smooth) OR Diabetic Jam						
	Morning tea (choose 1 option)						
	Plain Crackers & Cheese	Plain Crackers & Cheese	Plain crackers, cottage cheese	Plain crackers, cottage cheese	Plain Crackers and Cream Cheese	Plain Crackers & Cheese	Plain yogurt
	OR Plain or Digestive Biscuits (Graham Crackers) with Glass of Milk						
	LUNCH						
Soup	crème of tomato	Cream of Chicken	crème of tomato	Cream of Pumpkin	crème of tomato	Cream of Pumpkin	crème of tomato
	Sandwich (made with white or Wholemeal bread)						
Sandwich	Ham	Egg	Salmon	Ham	Beef	Ham	Egg
Extra	*Extra*						
Bakery	White Bread OR Wholemeal OR Rice Wafer						
Spreads	Margarine OR Butter with Peanut Butter (smooth) OR Diabetic Jam						
Fresh Fruit	Allowed Fruit						
	Afternoon tea (choose 1 option)						
	plain yogurt	Plain Crackers, Cream Cheese	plain yogurt	Plain Crackers, Cream Cheese	plain yogurt	Plain Crackers Cottage Cheese	Plain Crackers & Cheese
	OR Plain or Digestive Biscuits (Graham Crackers) with Milk						
	DINNER						
	Beef Curry with Rice and Spinach	Marinated Pork in Pita Bread	Chicken Chow Mein	Beef Casserole with Steamed Rice	Baked Fish in Coconut Cream with Mashed Potato, Spinach, Carrot	Silverbeet (Swiss Chard) Lamb Lasagna	Chicken Meatballs with Rice, Broccoli, Cauliflower & Parsley Sauce
Dessert	*Dessert (choose maximum of 2 Options)*						
	Custard (Sugar Free) with Diabetic Jelly						
	Pears – Stewed (drained)	Peaches – Stewed (drained)	Pears – Stewed (drained)	Peaches – Stewed (drained)	Apples - Stewed with Cinnamon	Pears – Stewed (drained)	Apples - Stewed with Cinnamon (dained)
	Supper						
Supper	plain Crackers & cream cheese	plain crackers, margarine, tuna	plain crackers, cottage cheese	plain crackers, margarine, tuna	plain crackers, cottage cheese	plain crackers, margarine, tuna	Plain Crackers & cream cheese
	with a glass of milk						

If needed for blood sugar control over night, can have a protein sandwich made with white bread for supper.

Shopping Lists

Shopping List - Week 1

Pantry Items

- ☐ Breadcrumbs
- ☐ Cornflour
- ☐ Flour
- ☐ Custard Powder
- ☐ Peanut Butter -smooth
- ☐ Nutmeg – ground
- ☐ Paprika - ground
- ☐ Rosemary – dried
- ☐ Black Pepper – ground
- ☐ Cumin – ground
- ☐ Salt
- ☐ Pepper – ground, black
- ☐ Pepper – ground, white
- ☐ Italian Herb Mix
- ☐ Hot drink options: tea, coffee, drinking chocolate etc.

- ☐ Tomato Sauce
- ☐ Worcestershire Sauce
- ☐ Ready made bolognaise sauce
- ☐ Tomato Paste
- ☐ Mayonnaise
- ☐ Garlic – to make garlic infused oil
- ☐ Onion – to make onion infused oil
- ☐ Honey
- ☐ Jam (or low sugar option)
- ☐ Sugar (not for those with diabetes)
- ☐ Clear Juice (apple, pear or orange) or get greens to make own green juices (see recipe section)
- ☐ Sugar free / Low sugar clear juice
- ☐ Olive Oil   2 Litres
- ☐ Margarine / butter   A tub
- ☐ Nutritional Yeast
- ☐ Diabetic Jelly (for diabetics)

Dairy / Eggs

- ☐ Milk — 2 L/1.2 gal
- ☐ Get extra milk for smoothies
- ☐ Egg — 1 dozen
- ☐ Cheese (plain) — a block
- ☐ Cottage Cheese — 1 x 250g/8oz
- ☐ Cream Cheese — 1 x 250g/8oz
- ☐ Plain Yogurt — 500g/18.8oz
- ☐ Ice-cream (for standard menu)
- ☐ Get extra yogurt for smoothies as needed.

Rice & Cereals

- ☐ Linguine Pasta — 170g/6oz
- ☐ Rice — 2 cups
- ☐ Tortilla Wrap — 4
- ☐ Cornflakes
- ☐ Fine Rolled Oats
- ☐ Rice Bubbles / Ricies/Rice Krispies
- ☐ Bread (white/wholemeal) 1-2 loaf/sliced
- ☐ Plain crackers — 2x packets
- ☐ Rice Waters — 1 packet
- ☐ Plain Biscuit or low sugar biscuit / Digestive Biscuits (Graham Crackers) (for diabetes) — 1 pack

Fruit & Vegetables

- ☐ Apricots, can, quartered — 100g/3oz
- ☐ Peaches – can, stewed — 3 cans
- ☐ Pears – can, stewed — 3 cans
- ☐ Apples – can, stewed — 3 cans
- ☐ Banana — 3-4 (not for those with diabetes)
- ☐ Avocado — 3 medium
- ☐ Beetroot - canned
- ☐ Broccoli — ½ head
- ☐ Carrot — 2 medium
- ☐ Cucumber — 1
- ☐ Lemon — 3
- ☐ Frozen Peas — 1 cup
- ☐ Potato — 1 medium
- ☐ Pumpkin — 100g/3.5oz
- ☐ Silverbeet — 100g/3.5oz
- ☐ Sweet Potato / Kumara — 1 medium
- ☐ —
- ☐ Get extra fruit/vegetables for the green juices / smoothies as needed

Shopping List - Week 1 Continued

Seafood & Meats

- ☐ Beef Mince — 2 x 200g/7oz
- ☐ Burger Buns — 2
- ☐ Diced boneless chicken — 200g/7oz
- ☐ Lamb Loin chips — 230g /½ lb
- ☐ Pork Shoulder Roast — 200g/7oz
- ☐ Prawn – shelled — 280g/10oz
- ☐ Salmon steak — 200g/7oz
- ☐ Canned Tuna / Salmon — 1 can (for those with Diabetes)
- ☐ Ham – shaved 60g/2oz for 1 servings of or 120g/4oz for 2 servings
- ☐ Chicken Deli cooked 60g/2oz for 1 servings of or 120g/4oz for 2 servings
- ☐ Beef sliced – Deli cooked 60g/2oz for 1 servings of or 120g/4oz for 2 servings

To make home made soup

Crème of Chicken Soup
- ☐ Diced Chicken — 340g/¾ lb
- ☐ Parsley — 1 large bunch
- ☐ Carrot — 2 large
- ☐ Potato — 1 large
- ☐ Chicken Broth — 1 cup
- ☐ Cream or Coconut Cream — ½ cup

Cream of Pumpkin Soup
- ☐ Pumpkin — 1 whole
- ☐ Chicken or Vegetable Broth — 1.5 L (3 x 4.5 oz packets)
- ☐ Cream — 500ml/14.5oz

Cream of Tomato
- ☐ Canned diced tomato — 1 can
- ☐ Chicken or Vegetable Broth — 1 cup

Shopping List - Week 2

Pantry Items

- ☐ Bay leaves — 1
- ☐ Cloves — 4
- ☐ Coriander Powder
- ☐ Turmeric powder
- ☐ Dried Basil
- ☐ Paprika Powder
- ☐ Cornflour
- ☐ Flour
- ☐ Mustard Sauce (seedless)
- ☐ Diabetic Jelly
- ☐ Ice Cream (for standard population)

Fruit & Vegetables

- ☐ Avocado — 3
- ☐ Broccoli — 1
- ☐ Potato — 4-6 medium
- ☐ Pumpkin — 1 large
- ☐ Carrot — 2 medium
- ☐ Sweet Potato / Kumara — 2 medium
- ☐ Swiss Chard / Silverbeet — 8 oz
- ☐ Lemon — 1
- ☐ Get extra fruit/vegetables for green juices and smoothies as needed.

Seafood & Meat

- ☐ Beef Mince — 220g/8oz
- ☐ Corned Beef / Silverside — 250g/9oz
- ☐ Diced Chicken — 220g/8oz
- ☐ Diced Shoulder Bacon (rind removed): 200g/7oz
- ☐ Lamb Shank — 2 shanks
- ☐ Scotch Fillet — 240g/8oz
- ☐ Fish Fillet — 2 Fillet (1 fillet = 120g/4oz)

Dairy / Eggs

- ☐ Cheese - grated
- ☐ Milk — 2L/1/2 Gal
- ☐ Eggs — ½ dozen
- ☐ yogurt — 500g/18.8oz

Rice & Cereals

- ☐ Dried Spaghetti — 120g/4oz

Check from last week if you need more of the following:

☐ Cornflakes ☐ Fine Rolled Oats ☐ Rice Bubbles / Ricies / Rice Krispies ☐ Bread (white, wholemeal) 1-2 loaf / sliced ☐ Plain crackers 2 x packets	☐ Margarine ☐ Butter ☐ Ham sliced 60g/2oz ☐ Rice Waters 1 packet ☐ Plain Biscuit or low sugar biscuit / Digestive Biscuits (Graham Crackers) (for diabetes) 1 packet

To make home made soup
 	
<u>Crème of Chicken Soup</u>
   ☐ Diced Chicken   340g / ¾ lb
   ☐ Parsley   1 large bunch
   ☐ Carrot   2 large
   ☐ Potato   1 large
   ☐ Chicken Broth   1 cup
   ☐ Cream or Coconut Cream ½ cup
<u>Cream of Pumpkin Soup</u>
   ☐ Pumpkin   1 whole
   ☐ Chicken or Vegetable Broth 1.5 L (3 x 4.5 oz packets)
   ☐ Cream   500ml/14.5oz
<u>Cream of Tomato</u>
   ☐ Canned diced tomato   1 can
   ☐ Chicken or Vegetable Broth 1 cup
	☐ Apricots, can, quartered 100g/3oz
	☐ Peaches – can, stewed 3 cans
	☐ Pears – can, stewed 3 cans
	☐ Apples – can, stewed 3 cans
	☐ Banana 3-4 medium
	(not for those with diabetes)

Shopping List - Week 3

Pantry Items

- [ ] Cardamon Pods — 2
- [ ] Cinnamon Stick — 3cm long
- [ ] Coriandar seeds — 2 Tb
- [ ] Dried Basil Leaves
- [ ] Fennel seed, ground
- [ ] Fennel seed — 1 tsp
- [ ] Ginger powder
- [ ] Star Anise — 1 flower
- [ ] Coconut Cream — 200g/7oz
- [ ] Diabetic Jelly
- [ ] Honey
- [ ] Oyster Sauce
- [ ] Sesane oil
- [ ] Soy sauce
- [ ] Tomato Pasata Sauce (strained pureed tomato) — 250g /8.8oz
- [ ] Kebab skewers — 4
- [ ] Ice cream (for standard menu)
- [ ] Custard powder

Fruit & Vegetables

- [ ] Avocado — 3
- [ ] Broccoli — 1
- [ ] Beetroot - sliced — 1 can
- [ ] Carrot — 8 medium
- [ ] Cauliflower — ½ head
- [ ] Lemon — 1
- [ ] Onion — 1
- [ ] Potato — 3 medium
- [ ] Swiss Chard / Silverbeet — 8 leaves
- [ ] Baby Spinach — 500g/18oz 5 cups
- [ ] Sweet potato / kumara — 1 medium

Rice & Cereals

- [ ] Chow Mein Noodles — 85g/3 oz
- [ ] Fresh Lasagna sheets — 3 sheets
- [ ] Pita Bread — 2 (6inch)
- [ ] Rice (basmati) — 500g/18oz

Seafood & Meat		**Dairy & Egg**	
☐ Beef strips or diced	220g/½ lb	☐ Cheese	
☐ Beef diced	220g/½ lb	☐ Milk	2L/1/2 gal
☐ Chicken drumsticks	4	☐ Egg	½ dozen
☐ Chicken Tenderloin or thighs	200g /6oz		
☐ Fish Fillet	200g/7oz) or 2 fillets		
☐ Lamb Mince	200g /7oz		
☐ Pork sirloin	220g/½ lb		

Check from last week if you need more of the following:

☐ Cornflakes ☐ Fine Rolled Oats ☐ Rice Bubbles / Ricies/Rice Krispies ☐ Bread (white, wholemeal) 1-2 loaf / sliced ☐ Plain crackers 2 x packets	☐ Margarine ☐ Butter ☐ Ham sliced: 60g/2oz or 120g/4oz ☐ Rice Waters 1 packet ☐ Plain Biscuit or low sugar biscuit / Digestive Biscuits (Graham Crackers) (for diabetes) 1 packet
To make home made soup <u>Crème of Chicken Soup</u> ☐ Diced Chicken 340g / ¾ lb ☐ Parsley 1 large bunch ☐ Carrot 2 large ☐ Potato 1 large ☐ Chicken Broth 1 cup ☐ Cream or Coconut Cream ½ cup <u>Cream of Pumpkin Soup</u> ☐ Pumpkin 1 whole ☐ Chicken or Vegetable Broth 1.5 L (3 x 4.5 oz packets) ☐ Cream 500ml/14.5oz <u>Cream of Tomato</u> ☐ Canned diced tomato 1 can ☐ Chicken or Vegetable Broth 1 cup	☐ Apricots, can, quartered 100g/3oz ☐ Peaches – can, stewed 3 cans ☐ Pears – can, stewed 3 cans ☐ Apples – can, stewed 3 cans ☐ Banana 3-4 medium (not for those with diabetes)

SECTION THREE
Recipes

Fruit Juice Recipes

(Including Green Juice)

Clear fruit juices especially those freshly juiced provide gut healing nutrients such as polyphenols that can help in preventing inflammation. They can also help provide those extra nutrients for the good microbiome, helping to maintain a healthy microbiome balance.

Just note that for clear fluid diet, free fluid diet and low roughage diet, these juices must not have any pulps. As you transition to a high fiber diet, you can easily convert these recipes into a smoothie which includes the fiber components. Your good gut bugs love these fibers.

You can add herbs and spices to these juices when appropriate. Turmeric, basil, mint, sage, oregano, rosemary etc. all have anti-bacterial, anti-inflammatory functions. Below are just some simple examples.

You can use apple or pineapple as the juice base and build your flavours from there on. Be daring.

Note, though, if you have burping or reflux, you may have SIBO (small bacterial intestinal overgrowth) or intestinal dysbiosis (wrong bugs growing in the wrong area of your gut). In that case, I suggest to either reduce the amount you are having or not have the specific juices that use fruit.

If you have diabetes, then watch for the sugar levels. Some of these juices may not be ideal for you (those using apple, pineapple, orange juice or beetroot for example).

These recipes are for one (1) serving.

Dandelion, Spinach, Cucumber, Celery Juice

Dandelion leaves -	6 - 8 leaves
Spinach leaves - chopped	½ cup
Cucumber - diced	1
Celery	4-6 stalk
Ginger - chopped	1 inch

Wash all your vegetables before juicing. Juice all ingredients together.

Spinach, Cucumber, Carrot, Green Apple Juice

Baby Spinach - chopped	1 cup

Green Grapes	20
Cucumber - diced	1
Carrot - scrabbed, chopped	1 medium
Granny Smith Apple - chopped	1
Green Pepper (optional) for zing!	½ (deseeded).

Wash all of these before chopping. Juice.

Celery, Broccoli, Orange, Cucumber Juice

Celery	4 stalks
Broccoli - florets	¼ broccoli
Orange	2
Cucumber	1

Wash, dice, chop, and juice!

Watermelon, Mint, Spinach Juice

Mint leaves	6 -8 depending on your taste
Watermelon	1 cup- chopped
Baby Spinach	½ cup

Wash mint leaves, and baby spinach leaves. Chop them. Add all the ingredients to the juicer and juice.

Basil, Coconut Water, Strawberry, Carrot Juice

Basil leaves - chopped	½ Tb
Coconut Water	1 cup
Strawberry - frozen	½ cup
Carrot - scrubbed and chopped	1 medium

Add all the ingredients to juicer, juice and drink.

Apple, Celery, Parsley, Ginger Juice

Apple	2
Celery	6 sticks
Parsley	1 bunch
Ginger	½ inch

Wash and dice apples, parsley, celery, and ginger. Add in juicer. Juice and drink.

Smoothie Recipes

Smoothies are a great way to get some nutrients in. Adding a protein powder to these smoothies can help in getting the needed protein into your diet.

If a smoothie is a meal replacement, aim to have around 25g to 30g of protein in a serving.

You can use three of these options to increase the protein amounts in your smoothie:

- Use of a Protein powder: this can be whey protein based or plant protein based (like pea protein isolate).
- Use of skim milk powder
- Use of Greek Yogurt or yogurt higher in protein. Use a low fat, low sugar option.

If you have diarrhea or sore tummy, you can replace the yogurt/milk with dairy free milk or yogurt but add in the pea protein isolate. It may be that your lactase enzyme (that breaks down cow's milk sugar lactose) is low due to infection / inflammation so going dairy free can help.

Note that these smoothies need to have minimum insoluble fiber for phase 2 of the plan. In the transition phase, you can blitz the smoothie into a smooth puree texture, keeping some of the fiber and in phase 4, you can add fiber. Though I caution against using small unbroken seeds or corn even in phase 4.

Also note, banana skin is a great prebiotic (food to grow probiotic bugs in our tummy) so in phase 3 and 4, you can add the banana skin (chop the ends of the banana) and rinse the outside of the skin with hot water and then add to the smoothie. It leaves a hairy feel in your mouth when drinking but you can get used to it.

Banana Pineapple Smoothie

Ingredients	Quantity	Method
Greek yogurt - low fat, low sugar	170g or 6oz	Put all in a jug or nutri-bullet and biltz.
Banana - Ripe	1 medium	
Pineapple Juice	1 cup	Pour into a glass and drink!
Skim Milk Powder	2 Tb	

Nutritional Analysis Per Serving

	USA	Australia	New Zealand
Energy (kJ/kCal)	1479 (353)	1507 (360)	1905 (455)
Protein (g)	25	23	24
Carbohydrate (g)	60	62	70
- Sugar (g)	54	53	64
Total Fat (g)	1.5	0.9	8.3
Sodium (mg)	88	140	155
Dietary fiber (g)	3.5	2.1	2.6
Insoluble fiber (g)	Not known	Not known	2

Mocha Smoothie

Ingredients	Quantity	Method
Milk, standard - cold	1 Cup	Put all in a jug or nutri-bullet and biltz.
Coffee - instant	1 tsp (may want more!)	
Skim milk powder or protein powder	2 Tb	Pour into a glass and drink!
Cocoa Powder	1 Tb (may want more)	

Nutritional Analysis Per Serving

	USA	Australia	New Zealand
Energy (kJ/kCal)	1207 (288)	1283 (307)	1328 (317)
Protein (g)	25	21	27
Carbohydrate (g)	14	33	16.5
- Sugar (g)	15	32	12.5
Total Fat (g)	15	10	16
- Saturated Fat (g)	6.3	6.5	9.8
Sodium (mg)	210	223	124
Dietary fiber (g)	7.7	2.3	2.3
Insoluble fiber (g)	Not known	Not known	2

Peanut Butter Smoothie

Ingredients	Quantity	Method
Greek yogurt - low fat, low sugar	170g or 6oz	Put all in a jug or nutri-bullet and blitz.
Banana - Ripe	1 medium	
Peanut Butter - smooth	2 Tb	Pour into a glass and drink!

For those without diabetes, you can add a teaspoon of honey for taste.

Nutritional Analysis Per Serving

	USA	Australia	New Zealand
Energy (kJ/kCal)	1669 (399)	1907 (456)	2119 (506)
Protein (g)	25	23	28
Carbohydrate (g)	31	38	33
- Sugar (g)	24	30	25
Total Fat (g)	19	20	29
- Saturated Fat (g)	5.3	5.4	9
Sodium (mg)	64	218	86
Dietary fiber (g)	4.6	8	7.9
Insoluble fiber (g)	Not known	Not known	Not known

Peachy Smoothie

Ingredients	Quantity	Method
Greek yogurt - low fat, low sugar	170g or 6oz	Put all in a jug or nutri-bullet and blitz.
Peaches, canned, drained	1 Cup	
Skim milk powder	1 Tb	Pour into a glass and drink!

For those without diabetes, you can add a teaspoon of honey for taste.

Nutritional Analysis Per Serving

	USA	Australia	New Zealand
Energy (kJ/kCal)	1283 (307)	1613 (386)	1631 (390)
Protein (g)	23	25	29
Carbohydrate (g)	30	48	39
- Sugar (g)	30	48	39
Total Fat (g)	4	5.8	13
- Saturated Fat (g)	2.5	3.5	7.5
Sodium (mg)	64	347	165
Dietary fiber (g)	3.7	10.2	3.2
Insoluble fiber (g)	Not known	Not known	Not known

Soup Recipes

These recipes are for 4 servings. You can always cool down extra soup and freeze it for later consumption. Remember to label your container with what it is and the date.

Crème of Chicken Soup

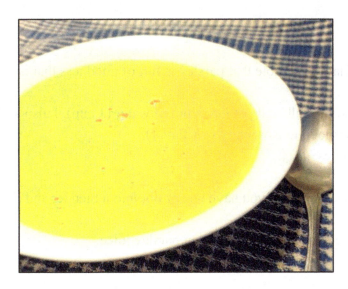

Ingredients	Quantity	Ingredients	Quantity
Garlic Infused Oil	1 Tb	Potatoes - peeled, diced	1 medium
Onion Infused Oil	1 Tb	Plain Flour	2 Tb
Diced Chicken Pieces (or tenderloin)	340g or ¾ pound	Chicken Broth	1 cup
Milk	2 cups	Cream (heavy) or Coconut Cream	½ cup
Parsley	1 large bunch	Water	1 cup
Carrot	2 large - diced	Salt & Pepper to taste	

Method

1. To make your own broth, in a pot, add four chicken frames to 3 cups of water, allow to boil and then turn own to slowly simmer for an hour to 90 minutes. Take off the stove.
2. Allow to cool down.
3. Pour out the broth into clean jug. Discard frame (unless there is meat on the frames, you can remove the meat to add to the soup).

A good quality broth made from chicken bones will have collagen in the water and that is great for gut healing.

Make Parsley Water

This is to give more flavor and note that parsley is full of goodness that is great for health and immunity.
1. Chop parsley including stalk and put into a pot of water (1 cup). I also added in 1 Tablespoon of Thyme and 1 Tablespoon to Rosemary (for flavor).
2. Simmer for 15 minutes.
3. Remove from the stove.
4. Use a handheld stick blender if you have one or put into a blender and blend to make a pureed liquid.
5. Once done, use a sieve and just get the green parsley juice.

Cooking Creme of Chicken
1. In a pot, heat the garlic infused oil and the onion infused oil, Add diced chicken pieces and lightly cook.
2. Add chicken broth, parsley water, diced carrots & diced pumpkin.
3. Cook in low heat for an hour, stirring occasionally.
4. Add salt & pepper to taste.
5. Check to see that the potato is cooked.
6. Remove pot from heat.
7. Use a stick blender to puree the soup to make creme of chicken soup.
8. Put back on stove to simmer.
9. Add cream, stir cream in and simmer for a few minutes.

Extra Ideas

I played with this above recipe to show how you can increase your options using the above recipe as a base idea.

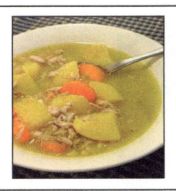	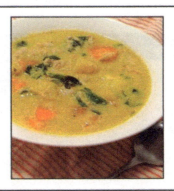	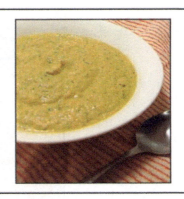
I did not puree the soup, left it with its component whole. My 11 year old liked this one the best as she said it had layers of flavour compared to the others.	In this one, I added sliced spinach (taking the stalks off first to decrease roughage). Tasted great to me but spinach had a slimy feel to it.	Pureed soup that had spinach in it. It tasted great and looked awesome too. But my 11 year old did not like it!

Nutritional Analysis Per Serving

	USA	Australia	New Zealand
Energy (kJ/kCal)	1696 (405)	1771 (423)	1680 (404)
Protein (g)	25	24.4	24
Carbohydrate (g)	19.6	21.8	17.5
- Sugar (g)	11.5	13	11
Total Fat (g)	25	26.6	26
Sodium (mg)	472	401	496
Dietary fiber (g)	1.3	1.1	0.9
Insoluble fiber (g)	Not known	Not known	0.72

Crème of Pumpkin Soup

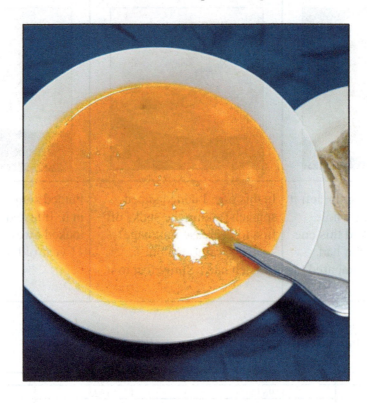

Ingredient	Quantity	Ingredient	Quantity
Pumpkin – deseeded	1kg or 2.2 lb	Nutmeg - ground	2 tsp
Garlic Crush	1 Tb (8cloves)	Cumin	2 tsp
Onion – diced	1 large	Salt & Pepper to taste	
Oil	3 Tb	Cream	½ cup
Chicken/Vegetable Stock or Broth	3 cups	Salt & Pepper to taste	
Water	1 cup		

Method

Prepare the base liquid.
1. In a large pot, heat oil.
2. Add onion and fry till onion is clear.
3. Add crushed garlic.
4. Simmer to cook until garlic is cooked.
5. Add vegetable/chicken stock and water to this.
6. Allow to simmer for 5 minutes.
7. Take pot off stove and run the liquid through a hand-held stick blender to finely puree all the onion/garlic mix through the mixture.
8. Put back on stove for 5 minutes and bring mixture to almost boiling temperature.

9. Remove pot from stove and run the liquid through a sieve to remove all the roughage. You can press out the liquid through the sieve and discard the left-over roughage.
10. Put liquid back in the pot and back on the stove.

Add in pumpkin

1. Cut pumpkin into large slice, remove skin and cut into 3 -3.5cm cubes.
2. Add pumpkin and simmer for 55 minutes until pumpkin is tender.
3. Remove from heat and use blender to puree the soup.
4. Add in cup of cream, salt, and pepper.

Ladle to serve.

Nutritional Analysis Per Serving

	USA	Australia	New Zealand
Energy (kJ/kCal)	1456 (348)	1116 (267)	1021 (244)
Protein (g)	8	6.4	3.4
Carbohydrate (g)	10.9	19	19.2
- Sugar (g)	1	13.9	12.9
Total Fat (g)	17.9	17.4	17.2
Sodium (mg)	281	689	1060
Dietary fiber (g)	1.3	1.1	3.4
Insoluble fiber (g)	Not known	Not known	0.5

Crème of Tomato Soup

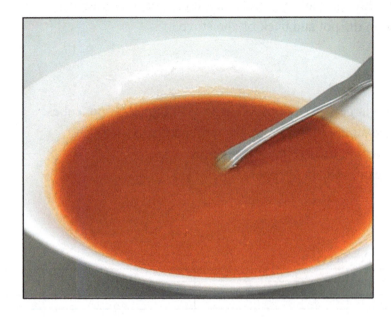

Ingredient	Quantity	Ingredient	Quantity
Canned Diced Tomato	1 can	Onion Infused Oil	1 Tb
Chicken or Vegetable Broth	1 cup	Cream	½ cup
Water	1 cup	Corn flour / Flour	1 Tb
Italian Herb Infused Oil	1 Tb	Sugar (optional)	1 Tb
Garlic Infused Oil	1 Tb	Salt & Pepper to taste	

Method

1. In a pot, add chicken or vegetable stock. Add in corn flour/flour for thickening. Whisk this in.
2. Add the oils and diced canned tomato to the pot. Add sugar (if need for a sweeter flavor but not for those with diabetes).
3. Allow to boil and then simmer for 10 minutes.
4. Take off stove.
5. Use a blender to puree.
6. Pass through sieve into a jug.
7. Add in cream.

Nutritional Analysis Per Servings

	USA	Australia	New Zealand
Energy (kJ/kCal)	1696 (405)	1771 (423)	1680 (401)
Protein (g)	25	24.4	24
Carbohydrate (g)	19.6	21.8	17.5
- Sugar (g)	11.5	13	11
Total Fat (g)	25	26.6	26
Sodium (mg)	472	401	496
Dietary fiber (g)	1.3	1.1	0.9
Insoluble fiber (g)	Not known	Not known	0.72

Adaptations For Vegan Diet

A vegan diet needs to meet its protein through use of nuts, seeds, lentils, legumes, beans, chickpeas, tempeh, tofu etc.

Since a low roughage diet means removing any harsh unbroken fibers, the following adaptations need to be made to meet the daily protein requirement:

1. Use smooth nut butter instead of nuts.

2. For lentils and legumes:

- use those that have no skin, such as red and yellow lentils.

- soak these overnight to allow the fibers to become softer with water. Remove water in the morning.

- smooth blend soups to ensure that every component is broken down.

- note that lentils, legumes etc. can cause bloating. Thus monitor the symptoms of bloating. It may be that your gut is unable to digest these at present.

3. Use tempeh and tofu as protein options. You could try marinating these overnight.

4. Chewing food till smooth in your mouth before swallowing is recommended.

5. Use protein powers like pea protein isolate where possible. Aim for 20g to 30g of protein for each meal.

Tofu (100g) has around 12g of protein.

Tempeh (100g) has 18g of protein.

Peanut butter (1Tb) has 3g of protein.

You can adapt some of the recipes given by substituting with a suitable plant protein option.

Dinner Recipes

These recipes are for two servings.

Week 1: Day 1: Citrus Salmon with Pea Puree with Mashed Sweet Potato

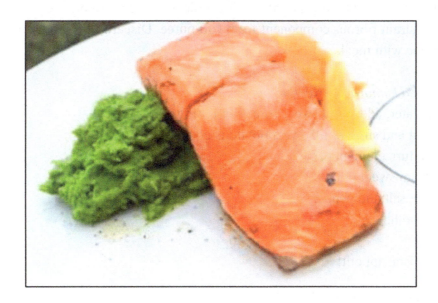

Ingredient	Quantity	Ingredient	Quantity
Garlic Infused Oil	1 Tb	Orange Juice	2 Tb
Onion Infused Oil	1 Tb	Salt, Table	1 dash
Salmon Steak	2 fillets (1 fillet: 100g/3.5 oz)	Peas	1 cup
		Sweet Potato, Peeled, Diced	1 medium size
Lemon Juice	1 lemon yield		2 Tb
Honey	1 Tb	Milk, Standard	1 heaped Tb
		Margarine	
		Salt & Pepper To Taste	

Method

1. In a bowl, mix garlic infused oil, onion infused oil, lemon juice, salt, and honey.
2. Heat a non-stick frying pan on medium heat.
3. Spray on oil.
4. Grill salmon with skin down for 10 – 15 minutes, basting with the marinade made above every 3 minutes. Turn over the last minute and grill off (however, you may not want to do that). Ensure that the salmon flakes with a fork.
5. Take of heat.
6. Serve with pureed peas and mashed potato.

To prepare pureed peas:
1. Defrost frozen peas.

2. Cook in boiling hot water till very soft.
3. Remove pan from heat. Drain water off. Using a blender, blend till pureed.
4. Using a sieve, strain fibrous component from soft puree. Discard fibrous residue.
5. Serve soft puree with meal.

To prepare mashed kumara or sweet potato
1. In a pot with water, add diced sweet potato and bring water to boil.
2. Turn down heat and simmer till sweet potato is cooked.
3. When cooked, turn element off.
4. Drain water from sweet potato.
5. Add margarine, salt and pepper, milk.
6. Mash until smooth.

Serve for dinner. Bon appétit!

Nutritional Analysis Per Serving

	USA	Australia	New Zealand
Energy (kJ/kCal)	2708 (647)	1970 (471)	2362 (565)
Protein (g)	28	21	24
Carbohydrate (g)	40	25	28
- Sugar (g)	26	15	14
Total Fat (g)	40	31.5	40
- Saturated Fat (g)	7.1	6.8	9.7
Sodium (mg)	1023	131	160
Dietary fiber (g)	5.5	4.3	3.0
Insoluble fiber (g)	Not known	Not known	2.7

Week 1: Day 2: Beef Burger

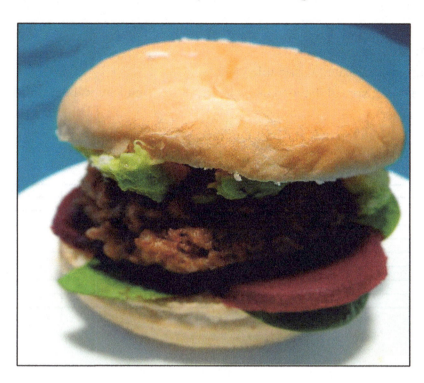

Ingredient	Quantity	Ingredient	Quantity
Olive Oil	2 Tb	Beetroot - canned, drained, dried	8 slices
Beef Mince	200g (7oz)	Baby Spinach	½ cup
Paprika	¼ tsp	Egg	1
Ground Cumin	¼ tsp	Flour	6 Tb
Avocado	½	Salt to taste	
Mayonnaise	2 Tb	Burger Buns	2

Method

To make mince patties.
1. In a bowl, add mince, egg, paprika, salt, cumin powder, and flour together and mix well.
2. Divide the mixture for two patties. Pat and shape in patty shapes.
3. Heat oil in a skillet / pan. Place patties on the pan and cook for 5 minutes on each side on low heat, checking to see that it is cooked. When cooked, put aside on a plate.

Prepare the salad component
1. Take of stalks of baby spinach.
2. Slice avocado into 8 slices
3. Use a paper towel to dry out the beetroot.

Prepare Beef Burger
1. Cut burger into half.
2. Lightly grill the exposed side of the burger for slight crunch.
3. Remove from being under a grill.
4. Place each burger on a plate to assemble.
5. On the bottom piece, spread mayonnaise, then layer spinach leaves, beetroot, beef patty, sliced avocado (4 per burger).
6. Cover with burger bun top half and eat! Dig in!

Nutritional Analysis Per Serving

	USA	Australia	New Zealand
Energy (kJ/kCal)	2768 (662)	2790 (667)	2495 (596)
Protein (g)	22	29	27
Carbohydrate (g)	17	51.7	51
- Sugar (g)	7.1	15.5	11
Total Fat (g)	55.7	36.3	34
- Saturated fat (g)	13	8	6.3
Sodium (mg)	468.9	794	657
Dietary fiber (g)	6.8	11	7.4
Insoluble fiber (g)	Not known	Not known	5.8

Week 1: Day 3: Apricot Chicken

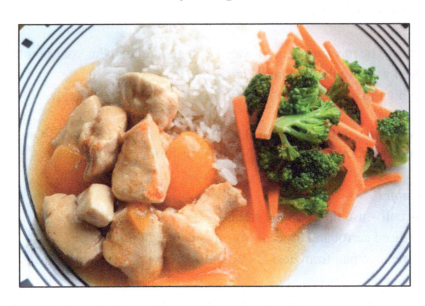

Ingredient	Quantity	Ingredient	Quantity
Diced Boneless Chicken	200g / 7oz	Tomato Sauce	1 Tb
Apricots, Canned, With Juice- Quartered	100g / 3.5 oz	Garlic Oil	2 Tb
		Rice	1 cup
Water	¼ cup	Broccoli	4 florets
Corn flour	2 Tb	Carrot, Peeled, Diced	1 large
Infused Onion Oil	2 Tb		
Salt Table	1 dash		

Method

To cook apricot chicken

1. Heat garlic oil and infused onion oil in a non-stick pan.
2. Add diced chicken and seal sides.
3. Add water, salt, tomato sauce and simmer for 10-15 minutes until the chicken is almost cooked.
4. Add apricots
5. Simmer for another 10 minutes.
6. If the liquid is too thin, add corn flour in a little bit of water and make a roux. Add to the chicken mix to thicken.
7. Simmer low for another 5 minutes. Turn off heat.

To cook rice in the microwave

1. Put rice in microwaveable dish
2. Wash 3 times.
3. Add water to rice. The measurement of water is done like this. Put your pointer finger to the top of the rice. Add water to the first knuckle.
4. Microwave on high for 9 minutes.
5. Take out and let it sit for 3 minutes.
6. Check that rice is cooked by pressing a flake in-between your finger and your thumb.
7. If still uncooked, add a bit more water and cook for further 2-3 minutes.

To prepare vegetables

1. Regarding broccoli – use tips, remove stems.
2. Steam or cook diced carrot and broccoli tips in a pan of boiling water.
3. When cooked, remove pan from heat, drain and serve with meal. Delicious!

Nutritional Analysis Per Serving

	USA	Australia	New Zealand
Energy (kJ/kCal)	1964 (469)	2650 (633)	3309 (794)
Protein (g)	25	29	31
Carbohydrate (g)	39	66	106
- Sugar (g)	2.1	9.1	12
Total Fat (g)	15.8	27	27
- Saturated Fat	1.5	3.3	3.3
Sodium (mg)	361	546	546
Dietary fiber (g)	3	7.3	4.7
Insoluble fiber (g)	Not known	Not known	1.6

Week 1: Day 4: Creamy Prawn Pasta

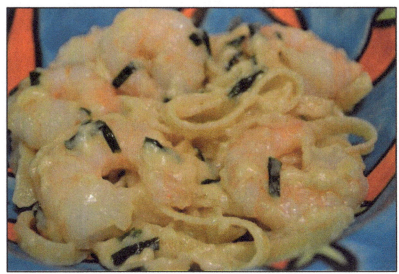

Ingredient	Quantity	Ingredient	Quantity
Prawn, Shelled	280g / 10oz	Whole Milk	½ cup
Garlic Oil	1 Tb	Ground Black Pepper	1 dash
Infused Onion Oil	1 Tb	Linguine pasta	170g / 6 oz
Corn flour	2 tsp	Lemon Juice	1 lemon yields

Method

1. Clean prawn to just flesh.
2. Cook linguini in a large saucepan of boiling, salted water according to packet directions. Add
3. peas 2 minutes before end of cooking time.
4. Drain and return to pan to keep warm.
5. Meanwhile, heat oil in a frying pan on high. Cook prawns, stirring for 2 minutes, until pink.
6. Stir in garlic, lemon juice. remove from heat.
7. In a separate pan, heat oil, make a roux using corn flour and milk.
8. Add prawn to this. Mix.
9. Pour over linguini. Mix.

Have a great meal!

Nutritional Analysis Per Serving

	USA	Australia	New Zealand
Energy (kJ/kCal)	1128 (270)	2189 (523)	1128 (370)
Protein (g)	21	35	21
Carbohydrate (g)	5.4	65	5.4
- Sugar (g)	3.9	1.9	3.9
Total Fat (g)	13	40g	13
- Saturated Fat	2.4	13	2.4
Sodium (mg)	841	509	841
Dietary fiber (g)	0.5	2.8	0.5
Insoluble fiber (g)	Not known	Not known	Not known

Week 1: Day 5: Braised Lamb Chop with Rice

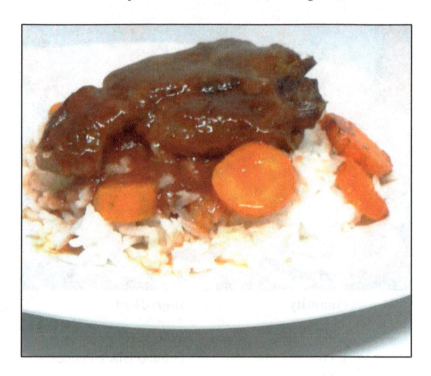

Ingredient	Quantity	Ingredient	Quantity
Rice	½ cup	Lamb Loin Chops	230g / ½ pound
Garlic Oil	1 Tb	Tomato Paste	2 Tb
Rosemary Leaves, Dried	1 tsp.	Water	4 Tb
Water	2 Tb	Lemon Juice	1 lemon yields
Carrot	1 large		

Method

Preheat oven at 150°C/300°F

Cook rice in the microwave
1. Put rice in microwaveable dish,
2. Wash 3 times.
3. Add 1 cup water to rice.
4. Microwave on high for 10 minutes.
5. Take out and let it sit for 3 minutes.
6. Check that the rice is cooked by pressing a flake in-between your finger and your thumb.
7. If still uncooked, add a bit more water and cook for further 2-3 minutes.

Cook braised lamb chop

1. Pound rosemary to remove juice from leaves.
2. Once the juice has separated from leave, add 2 tsp of water and mix.
3. Pour mixture through a sieve to remove all debris and roughage.
4. In a cup, mix tomato paste, rosemary juice, water, and corn flour.
5. In a casserole dish, pour garlic infused oil and onion infused oil.
6. Lay lamb chops in the casserole dish. Lay carrot on top. And pour the tomato mix on top.
7. Bake for 45 minutes. Check to see that the meat is cooked.
8. Serve with steamed rice.

Relish every bite!

Nutritional Analysis Per Serving

	USA	Australia	New Zealand
Energy (kJ/kCal)	1895 (453)	2485	3811 (911)
Protein (g)	27	28	30
Carbohydrate (g)	39	28	85.6
- Sugar (g)	5.1	9.1	5.1
Total Fat (g)	19	33	50.1
- Saturated Fat	4.2	13	19.2
Sodium (mg)	312	116	92
Dietary fiber (g)	4.2	3.5	3.3
Insoluble fiber (g)	Not known	Not known	1.9

Week 1: Day 6: Beef Meatball in Tortilla Wrap with Cucumber, Carrot

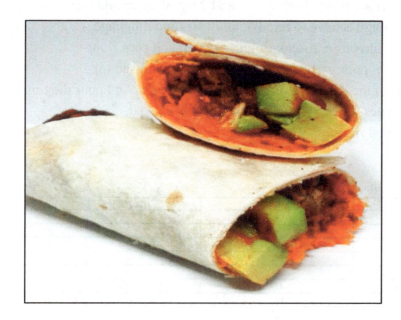

Ingredient	Quantity	Ingredient	Quantity
Olive Oil	4 Tb	Worcestershire Sauce	1 tsp
Beef Mince – Lean	200g / 7 oz	Salt	To taste
Bread Crumbs – Dry	3 Tb	Ready Made Bolognaise Sauce	½ can (100g / 3.5 oz)
Garam Masala	¾ tsp	Tortilla Wrap – Ready Made	2
Nutmeg- Ground	½ tsp	Cucumber (Deseeded, Peeled)	½ medium cucumber
White Pepper	½ tsp	Carrot	1 medium size
Onion Infused Oil	1 tsp	Avocado	½ medium size
Garlic Infused Oil	1 tsp		

Method

To make meatballs

1. Mix all ingredients (except the sunflower oil) together.
2. Roll into 20g balls – makes 12 balls.
3. Place on a tray.
4. Heat sunflower oil in frying pan.
5. Gently put each meatball in the frying pan and cook under low heat, turning regularly to ensure even cooking.
6. When cooked, remove, and put on clean plate.

Bolognaise sauce: need a sieve.

I used readymade bottled bolognaise sauce.

1. Pour bolognaise sauce through a sieve to remove all big particles, to collect a smooth sauce in a bottom container.
2. Discard all the sieved particles.
3. In a pot, heat the sieved bolognaise sauce.
4. Add the cooked lamb meatballs to the sauce and simmer for 5 minutes in low heat.

Prepare the tortilla meal

1. Place a tortilla wrap on plate.
2. Layer across grated carrot, sliced cucumber, take 5 meatballs and put side by side length wise on the vegetable layer.
3. Add sliced avocado on top.
4. Roll the side of the wrap together to encase.
5. Cut across in half in the center.

Wishing you a tasty meal!

Nutritional Analysis Per Serving

	USA	Australia	New Zealand
Energy (kJ/kCal)	2328 (556)	2167 (518)	2078 (497(
Protein (g)	29	30	26.7
Carbohydrate (g)	29	47	30.2
- Sugar (g)	4	9.7	4.5
Total Fat (g)	28	22	30.3
- Saturated Fat	4.4	6	5.6
Sodium (mg)	1147	572	168
Dietary fiber (g)	7.6	7.2	7.5
Insoluble fiber (g)	Not known	Not known	5.7

Week 1: Day 7: Roast Pork, Mashed Potato, Boiled Pumpkin, Silverbeet / Swiss Chard

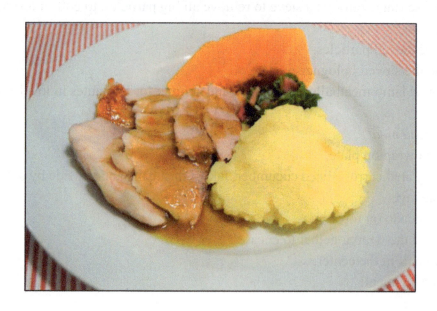

Ingredient	Quantity	Ingredient	Quantity
Olive Oil	1 Tb	Pumpkin	100g / 3.5 oz
Pork Shoulder Roast	200g	Silverbeet	100g / 3.5 oz
Salt	Pinch	Milk	2 Tb
Potato, Diced	1 medium	Margarine /Butter	1 Tb
Salt & Pepper to Taste.			

Method

Pre-heat oven to 205°C/400°F

1. Place pork shoulder roast on rack in a roasting dish. Rub salt on the skin.
2. Roast for 15 minutes. Reduce temperature to 150°C/300°F and roast further for 45 minutes.
3. Pork is cooked when internal temperature reaches at least 71°C/160°F
4. Remove from oven and set aside to rest.
5. Boil diced potatoes.
6. In separate pots, boil pumpkin and silver beet. When cooked, drain off water.
7. Drain and mash with milk and margarine.
8. Season with salt and pepper.

Here's to good food and good company!

Nutritional Analysis Per Serving

	USA	Australia	New Zealand
Energy (kJ/kCal)	1353 (323)	1001 (239)	1001 (239)
Protein (g)	17	23	23
Carbohydrate (g)	18	16	16.1
- Sugar (g)	0.3	3	56
Total Fat (g)	24	9g	3
- Saturated Fat	8.5	3	9.1
Sodium (mg)	1681	404	404
Dietary fiber (g)	3.2	3	3.4
Insoluble fiber (g)	Not known	Not known	1.5

Week 2: Day 1: Scotch Fillet, Mashed Potato with Steamed Pumpkin & Broccoli

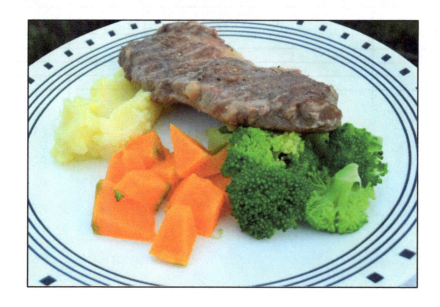

Ingredient	Quantity	Ingredient	Quantity
Scotch Fillet	240g	Margarine / Butter	1 Tb
Olive Oil	1 tsp	Salt	To taste
Salt	Dash	Pumpkin	100g
Potato, Peeled	160g	Broccoli	6 florets
Milk	1 Tb		

Method

Cook scotch fillet
1. Heat oil in non-stick pan on high heat.
2. Rub salt on the scotch fillet and cook as follows: cook 2 minutes each side for rare, 3-4 mins each side for medium-rare and 4-6 mins each side for medium. For well done, cook for 2-4 minutes each side, then turn the heat down and cook for another 4-6 minutes.
3. When cooked, remove, cover with foil and rest for a few minutes (5-7 minutes), remove foil, cut and serve.

To prepare the vegetables
1. Boil diced potato in water until soft. Drain water off when cooked.
2. Mash potato with milk, margarine/butter and salt until smooth.

3. Similarly boil peeled diced pumpkin until soft, drain water off when cooked.

4. Steam or boil broccoli tips. Drain water.

5. Plate up.

Hope it hits the spot!

Nutritional Analysis Per Serving

	USA	Australia	New Zealand
Energy (kJ/kCal)	1549 (370)	1351 (323)	1549 (370)
Protein (g)	36	38	36
Carbohydrate (g)	18	14	18
- Sugar (g)	1.2	3.7	1.2
Total Fat (g)	16	12	16
- Saturated Fat	4.9	3.8	4.9
Sodium (mg)	343	347	343
Dietary fiber (g)	4.2	3.4	4.2
Insoluble fiber (g)	Not known	Not known	Not known

Week 2: Day 2: Bacon Egg Potato Top Pie

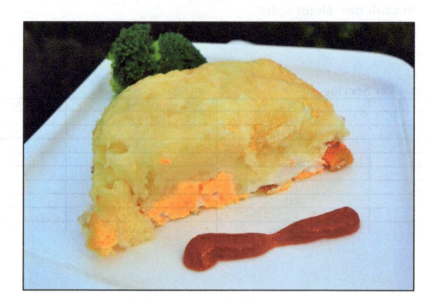

Ingredient	Quantity	Ingredient	Quantity
Diced Shoulder Bacon Pieces (Remove Rind)	200g / 7 oz	Whole Milk	3 Tb
Whole Egg	4 small eggs	Ground Black Pepper	1 dash
Ground White Pepper	¼ tsp	Grated Cheese	60g or 2 oz
Steamed Diced Carrot	1/2 cup	Tomato Sauce	4 Tb
Peeled Diced Medium Potato	170g / 6 oz	Broccoli tip	1 large floret

Method

1. Boil and mash diced potato. Add milk, seasonings to taste.
2. Turn oven to 180°C/350°F
3. In a small flan dish, place steamed diced carrot
4. Break whole egg on the mixed vegetable.
5. Add ground white pepper to taste
6. Layer mashed potato on top.
7. Sprinkle cheese on top
8. Place in oven and cook for 20 minutes, checking in the end with a knife prick to see that the egg is cooked. If it is not, cook for another 5-10 minutes.
9. Remove from the oven when cooked, slice and serve hot.

Take your time and enjoy!

Nutritional Analysis Per Serving

	USA	Australia	New Zealand
Energy (kJ/kCal)	2975 (711)	1776 (424)	4076 (974)
Protein (g)	30	28	26
Carbohydrate (g)	22.7	19.7	15.7
- Sugar (g)	5.7	2	2
Total Fat (g)	52	24	91
- Saturated Fat	19.6	11.9	38.3
Sodium (mg)	1279	1053	828
Dietary fiber (g)	4	9.6	1.6
Insoluble fiber (g)	Not known	Not known	0.3

Week 2: Day 3: Moroccan Lamb Shank with Sweet Potato or Kumara, Swiss Chard/Silverbeet, Pumpkin

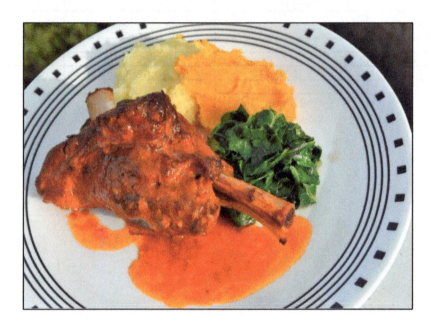

Ingredient	Quantity	Ingredient	Quantity
Garlic Oil	1 Tb	Salt	Dash
Infused Onion Oil	1 Tb	Water	1 cup
Lamb Shank	2 shanks	Potato, Medium, Peeled	200g / 7 oz
Ground Cumin Seed	½ tsp	Milk, Standard	4 Tb
Coriander Powder	½ tsp	Swiss Chard / Silverbeet	140g / 5 oz
Turmeric	1 tsp	Pumpkin (Skinless, Seedless, Diced)	120g / 4 oz
Tomato paste	3 Tb		

Method

To prepare mashed potato
1. Boil diced potato till soft.
2. Drain off water.
3. Mash with milk and add seasoning

To cook Moroccan Lamb Shank
1. Heat infused oil in a frying pan.
2. Seal the lamb shank to intensify taste. Remove from heat.
3. In a bowl, mix tomato paste, tomato paste, coriander powder, turmeric, and water.
4. Turn on a slow cooker to high. Add lamb shank, pour tomato mix on this. Add salt to taste

5. Slow cook for 4-6 hours, turning the lamb shank couple of times during this period.

To prepare vegetables
1. Take required amount of Silverbeet/Swiss chard. Remove soft leafy part from white stalk.
2. Add to a pot of boiling water. Simmer till soft. Drain and serve with meal.
3. Boil pumpkin till soft. Drain and serve with meal. When cooked, serve with rice.

Hope it's as delicious as it looks!

Nutritional Analysis Per Serving

	USA	Australia	New Zealand
Energy (kJ/kCal)	2690 (643)	2280 (545)	2141 (512)
Protein (g)	49	39	49
Carbohydrate (g)	27	34	28
- Sugar (g)	8.8	10.4	13
Total Fat (g)	26	26	22
- Saturated Fat	6.6	8.2	5
Sodium (mg)	1182	671	1182
Dietary fiber (g)	7	8.4	5.2
Insoluble fiber (g)	Not known	Not known	2.1

Week 2: Day 4: Pan Fried Fish with Lemon Slice, Mashed Potato, Broccoli

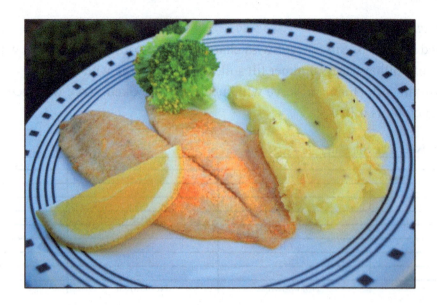

Ingredient	Quantity	Ingredient	Quantity
Fish Fillet	2 fillets (1 fillet: 120g or 4 oz)	Salt, Table	½ tsp
Olive Oil	1 Tb	Lemon Slice	4 wedges
Flour	4 Tb	Potato, Peeled	1 medium (200g/ 7oz)
Ground Cumin	¼ tsp	Milk, Standard	2 Tb
Paprika Powder	¼ tsp	Salt	Dash
Ground Coriander	¼ tsp	Ground Pepper	Dash
		Broccoli Tip	140g

Method

To cook fish fillet
1. Mix flour, paprika, cumin, coriander together.
2. Coat fish fillet with the flour mixture.
3. Heat oil in shallow fry pan. Pan fry for few minutes on each side, to cook and seal the fish. Should have a reddish golden coating.
4. Remove from pan and servings of with lemon wedges with vegetables

To prepare the vegetables
1. Boil peeled diced potato till soft. Drain off water, add salt, milk and ground pepper and mash till smooth.
2. Boil broccoli tip. When cooked, drain off water.
Treat yourself to this!

Nutritional Analysis Per Serving

	USA	Australia	New Zealand
Energy (kJ/kCal)	1159 (227)	1534 (367)	2153 (514)
Protein (g)	23	27	32
Carbohydrate (g)	18	40	40
- Sugar (g)	1.3	2.6	3
Total Fat (g)	10	12	25
- Saturated Fat	1.7	2	6
Sodium (mg)	435	627	578
Dietary fiber (g)	5.2	4.6	4.1
Insoluble fiber (g)	Not known	Not known	2.2

Week 2: Day 5: Chicken in Basil Sauce

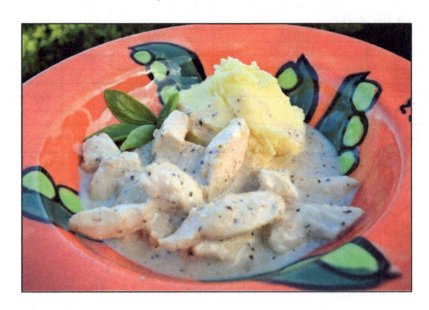

Ingredients	Quantity	Ingredients	Quantity
Margarine	1 Tb	Diced Chicken	220g/8oz
Corn Flour	2 tsp	Infused Garlic Oil	1 tsp
Milk	100 mL	Infused Onion Oil	2 tsp
Ground Dried Basil	1 Tb	Potato, Peeled Diced	2 x medium (200g/7oz)

Method

1. Heat infused oil in saucepan.
2. Brown diced chicken. Simmer at low heat.
3. Heat margarine in a pot and make a roux with corn flour and a small amount of milk.
4. Add the rest of the milk, stirring regularly to make a smooth sauce.
5. Add ground dried basil.
6. Add to the browned chicken and allow to simmer to cook chicken.
7. When cooked, remove from heat and servings of with mashed potato or steamed rice and low roughage seasonal vegetables

Have a great meal!

Nutritional Analysis Per Serving

	USA	Australia	New Zealand
Energy (kJ/kCal)	2821 (674)	1420 (33)	1681 (401)
Protein (g)	27	28	29
Carbohydrate (g)	75	19.6	22
- Sugar (g)	3.2	2.8	2.6
Total Fat (g)	21	15.8	22
- Saturated Fat	4.9	2.9	4.9
Sodium (mg)	1376	407	455
Dietary fiber (g)	8.3	1.8	2.5
Insoluble fiber (g)	Not known	Not known	0.8

Week 2: Day 6: Spaghetti Bolognaise with Broccoli

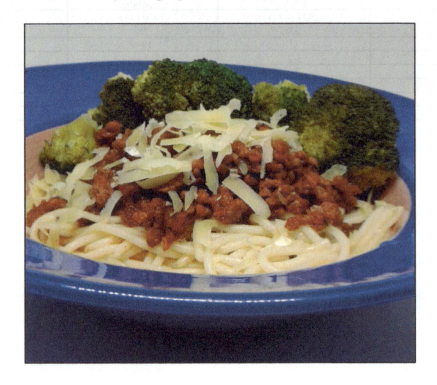

Ingredients	Quantity	Ingredients	Quantity
Tomato Paste	4 Tb	Onion Infused Oil	1 Tb
Beef Mince	220g or 8 oz	Spaghetti, Dried	120g or 4 oz
Ground Cumin Seed	1 Tb	Grated Cheese	40g or 1.5oz
Salt Table	1 dash	Broccoli Floret	2 florets
Garlic infused Oil	1 Tb		

Method

To cook Bolognaise
1. Add the tomato paste into a strainer and remove all seeds and skins etc.
2. Heat garlic infused oil and onion infused oil in a non-stick frying pan.
3. Brown beef mince.
4. Add the crushed tomato liquid and allow to simmer down using low heat.
5. Mix ground cumin.
6. Add salt to taste.
7. Remove from heat.

To cook Spaghetti
1. In a large pan, boil water

2. Add spaghetti to water
3. Boil for 12 minutes.
4. Drain off water.
5. Serve with bolognaise.
6. Add grated cheese on top before serving.

Delicious!

Nutritional Analysis Per Serving

	USA	Australia	New Zealand
Energy (kJ/kCal)	2116 (506)	1989 (475)	2040 (488)
Protein (g)	35	33	39
Carbohydrate (g)	36	71	43
- Sugar (g)	4.7	2	3.2
Total Fat (g)	23	17.9	17.5
- Saturated Fat	6.3	6.1	7
Sodium (mg)	763	341	268
Dietary fiber (g)	3.1	8.2	4.8
Insoluble fiber (g)	Not known	Not known	2

Week 2: Day 7: Corned Silverside, Sweet Potato, Carrot, Silverbeet/Swiss Chard

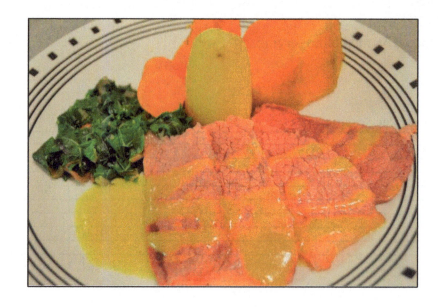

Ingredients	Quantity	Ingredients	Quantity
Corned Silverside	250g / 9 oz	Sweet Potato / Kumara	200g or 7oz
Malt Vinegar	2 Tb	Pumpkin	80g or 3 oz
Bay Leaves	1	Swiss Chard / Silverbeet	80g or 3 oz
Cloves	4	Ready Made – Seedless Mustard Sauce	½ cup
Water	2 cups		

Method

1. In a slow cooker, place corned silverside.
2. Add malt vinegar, cloves, and bay leaf to this.
3. Cover in water.
4. Cook on high for 4 – 6 hours until meat is tender.
5. Remove bay leaf and cloves.
6. Peel and dice pumpkin and kumara.
7. Place in boiling water and cook till soft.
8. When preparing Silverbeet (Swiss chard), just remove the green leaves from white stalk.
9. Boil in water till leaves are soft and cooked.
10. When the corned silverside is ready, slice for service.

Enjoy!

Nutritional Analysis Per Serving

	USA	Australia	New Zealand
Energy (kJ/kCal)	2233 (533)	1360 (325)	2081 (497)
Protein (g)	41	23	21
Carbohydrate (g)	4	22	64
- Sugar (g)	0	11	16
Total Fat (g)	18	15	18
- Saturated Fat	5.8	6.8	6.1
Sodium (mg)	1483	814	1799
Dietary fiber (g)	3.4	4.4	4
Insoluble fiber (g)	Not known	Not known	2

Week 3: Day 1: Beef Curry, Rice, and Spinach

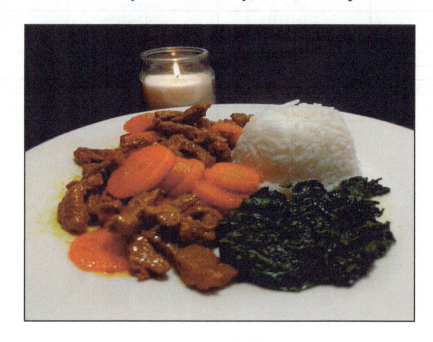

Ingredient	Quantity	Ingredient	Quantity
Olive Oil	7 Tb	Turmeric	1 tsp
Cardamon Pods	2	Beef strips or diced	220g (½ pound)
Cinnamon Stick	3 cm long	Carrot - sliced round	2 large
Coriander Seed	2 Tb	Spinach	12 large leaves
Star Anise	1 flower	Rice	½ cup
Garlic	2 cloves	Onion - fine diced	½ onion
Water	½ cup	Corn flour	1 Tb

Method

In this recipe, I tried a different method to see if I can produce a delicious low roughage beef curry from scratch. It works, deliciously.

To cook the beef curry
1. In a mortar, add garlic, cardamon, cinnamon stick, coriander seeds, star anise. Using mortar, crush into fine powder.
2. In a pot, add 3 Tb of the oil. Sauté onion until it is clear.
3. Add the garlic paste to this. On low heat for a minute, until the garlic looks crisp.
4. Add the 2 Tb of oil to this. Remove from heat.
5. Put another pot on stove, on medium heat.
6. Pour the mixture onto a sieve that is held above the second pot on the stove.

7. Use a teaspoon and press through the oil from the rough fried mixture into the second pot. The oil is now infused with all the spices.
8. Add turmeric to this.
9. Add diced or stripped beef into the second pot. Stir the beef to coat the beef pieces with the spices.
10. Add sliced carrots to this.
11. Add ½ cup water to this and mix through.
12. Allow to simmer on low heat for 10 minutes.
13. When cooked, mix corn flour in couple of tablespoons of curried liquid from the beef curry.
14. Add to the beef curry and simmer further for another 10 minutes to cook the beef and carrot.
15. When cooked, turn off the stove and put aside for service.

Cook rice in the microwave
1. Put rice in microwaveable dish,
2. Wash 3 times.
3. Add 1 cup water to rice.
4. Microwave on high for 10 minutes.
5. Take out and let it sit for 3 minutes.
6. Check that the rice is cooked by pressing a flake in-between your finger and your thumb.
If still uncooked, add a bit more water and cook for further 2-3 minutes.

To light fry the spinach
1. Remove stem from the spinach as discussed in Chapter 4.
2. Slice spinach leaves into thin strips.
3. Heat remaining 2 Tb of oil in a pot.
4. Add sliced spinach to this.
5. Add salt and stir to cook.
6. When spinach has been lightly fried, serve with beef curry and rice.
Like they say in Hindi – Saward! (Delicious!)

Nutritional Analysis Per Serving

	USA	Australia	New Zealand
Energy (kJ/kcal)	3047 (7289	2776 (663)	3555 (850)
Protein (g)	28	34	29
Carbohydrate (g)	22	49	53
- Sugar (g)	5	5.6	6.3
Total Fat (g)	57.9	34	58
- Saturated Fat	10.1	6.0	11
Sodium (mg)	164	110	102
Dietary fiber (g)	7	10.3	7.7
Insoluble fiber (g)	Not known	Not known	Not known

Week 3: Day 2: Marinated Pork Kebab With Pita Bread

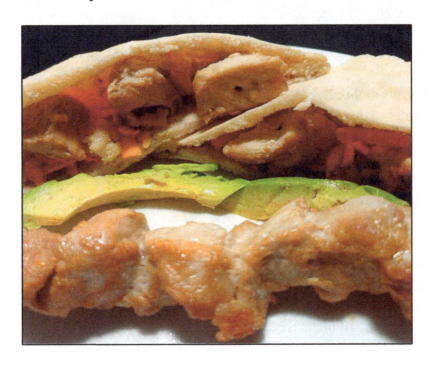

Ingredient	Quantity	Ingredient	Quantity
Garlic - crushed	1 Tb	Pork Sirloin	220g (½ pound)
Soy Sauce - low salt	¼ cup	Cauliflower	½ medium sized
Honey	2 Tb	Carrot (medium size)	2
Ginger - Powder	½ tsp	Avocado	½
Sesame Oil	1 Tb	Pita Bread- wholemeal	2 (6-inch size)
Kebab Skewers	4	Salt & Pepper to taste	

Method

To prepare pork kebab
1. Cut pork sirloin into 2cm cubes.
2. Prepare soy sauce marinate: in a bowl, add soy sauce, ginger powder, crushed garlic, and honey and mix well.
3. Put the pork sirloin cubes into the marinate, mix through, covering the pork cubes. Leave in covered bowl for 20 minutes.
4. After 20 minutes, divide the cubes into equal amounts for 4 kebab skewers. Push pork cubes through kebab skewers to make a pork kebab. Brush off any crushed garlic that might stick to the pork.

5. Either on a BBQ or in a frying pan, cook the pork kebab: couple of minutes on each side. You can brush on the marinate on the kebab halfway through the cooking to give it moisture and stickiness. Be careful not to cause the pork to burn (honey is both sticky and can caramelize).
6. When cooked, remove pork kebab from heat and put on a clean plate. Cover this.

To prepare the vegetable fillings
1. Cut the florets of the cauliflower (removing the stems) and divide the florets into smaller florets.
2. Peel and grate the carrot in a bowl.
3. Slice avocado into 4-6 slices (depending on the size of the avocado).
4. Heat a wok or skillet. Add some oil to this.
5. Lightly fry the cauliflower florets.
6. Add salt to taste. When cooked, put aside.

Prepare to fill the pita bread.
1. Cut pita bread into half.
2. Open the pita pocket and fill it with cauliflower and carrot.
3. Remove half of the pork from the kebab skewer and put into the pocket.

Before eating, add the avocado into the pocket, to give the fillings a moist feel. Enjoy eating.

Nutritional Analysis Per Serving

	USA	Australia	New Zealand
Energy (kJ/kCal)	1738 (415)	2528 (604)	2302 (550)
Protein (g)	34.6	38	34
Carbohydrate (g)	26	66	53.7
- Sugar (g)	24.7	35.8	19.2
Total Fat (g)	17.6	17.9	21.4
- Saturated Fat	1.9	3.1	3.7
Sodium (mg)	1671	1650	1650
Dietary fiber (g)	10.7	14.9	9.7
Insoluble fiber (g)	Not known	Not known	6.5

Week 3: Day 3: Chicken Chow Mein

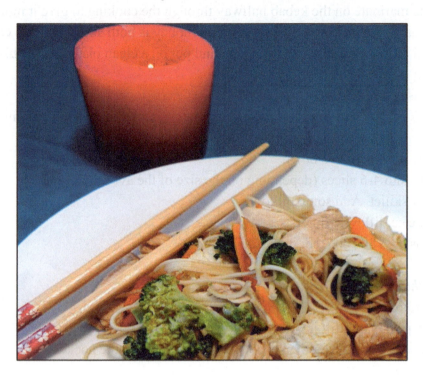

Ingredient	Quantity	Ingredient	Quantity
Chicken Tenderloins or Thigh	200g (6 oz)	Chow Mein Sauce	
Onion Infused Oil	1 Tb	Soy Sauce – low salt	1 ½ Tb
Garlic Infused Oil	1 Tb	Oyster Sauce	1 ½ Tb
Cauliflower	4 florets	Sesame Oil	½ Tb
Carrot (medium size)	2	Corn flour	2 tsp
Broccoli	4 florets	White Pepper	To taste
Chow Mein Noodles	85g (3 oz)	Water	½ cup

Method

Make the sauce
In a bowl, add all the sauce ingredients together and put to side.

Prepare the vegetables
1. Prepare the florets of cauliflower and broccoli: each floret can be cut into 4 slices or you can slice them too.
2. Julienne cut carrots (3 inch in length).

Prepare the chicken & noodles

1. Slice chicken tenderloin or thigh to 3-inch slices. I prefer to use tenderloin or thigh as it is moister compared to the chicken breast which can be dryer.
2. Pour the Chow Mein sauce onto this, mix to coat the chicken and put aside for 10 minutes.
3. In a wok or pan, heat garlic and onion infused oil.
4. Add the marinated chicken meat (not the sauce) to the wok and cook to make a tinged color (but not fully cook inside).
5. Add the vegetables to this and cook for 2 minutes, stirring occasionally. Vegetables should remain crunchy.
6. Add Chow Mein noodles to the wok.
7. Add the leftover sauce.
8. Stir fry for couple of minutes till the noodles are cooked. Use a pair of tongs to separate the chow mein noodles. (Alternatively, you can cook the chow mein noodles in a separate pot of boiling water. When cooked au dente, drain out the hot water. Then rinse under cold water. Then add to the chicken vegetable mix above).

Remove from heat and serve.

"吃得开心" = Enjoy your meal

Nutritional Analysis Per Serving

	USA	Australia	NZ
Energy kj/kcal	2264 (541)	2072 (459)	2494 (596)
Protein (g)	24	29	32
Carbohydrate (g)	40	50	72.2
- Sugar (g)	4.5	6.6	13.7
Fat (g)	35	18	19.6
- Saturated Fat	6.6	3.1	3.5
Sodium (mg)	1417	1386	654
Dietary fiber (g)	4.5	6.2	5.7
Insoluble fiber (g)	Not known	Not known	3.2

Week 3: Day 4: Beef Casserole

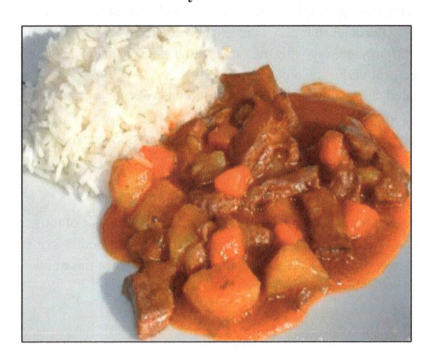

Ingredient	Quantity	Ingredient	Quantity
Garlic Oil	1 Tb	Paprika	1 tsp
Infused Onion Oil	1 Tb	Corn flour	1 Tb
Diced Beef	200g	Carrots diced	1 medium
Water	½ cup	Potatoes, Peeled, Diced	2 (120g/ 4.2 oz
Worcestershire Sauce	2 tsp	Salt, Table	2 dashes
		Rice, Basmati	1 cup

Method

1. Heat garlic infused oil and onion infused oil on a non-stick frying pan.
2. Add diced beef and sauté to seal the meat. Remove from heat.
3. In a crock pot, add all the rest of the ingredients except corn flour. Add sealed diced beef
4. Slow cook for 6 hours.
5. Stir in corn flour in the liquid component.
6. Slow cook for another hour or two.

To cook rice in the microwave
1. Put rice in microwaveable dish,
2. Wash 3 times.

3. Add water to rice. The measurement of water is done like this. Put your pointer finger to the top of the rice. Add water to the first knuckle.

4. Microwave on high for 9 minutes.

5. Take out and let it sit for 3 minutes.

6. Check that rice is cooked by pressing a flake in-between your finger and your thumb.

7. If still uncooked, add a bit more water and cook for further 2-3 minutes.

Let's eat and enjoy!

Nutritional Analysis Per Serving

	USA	Australia	New Zealand
Energy (kJ/kCal)	2062 (493)	1632 (390)	2494 (835)
Protein (g)	26	27	37
Carbohydrate (g)	56	30	110
- Sugar (g)	6.7	9.4	56
Total Fat (g)	16	17g	27
- Saturated Fat	3.5	3.3	7.8
Sodium (mg)	416	771	6346
Dietary fiber (g)	6.5	7	3.4
Insoluble fiber (g)	Not known	Not known	1.3

Week 3: Day 5: Fish Baked In Coconut Cream, Sweet Potato & Spinach

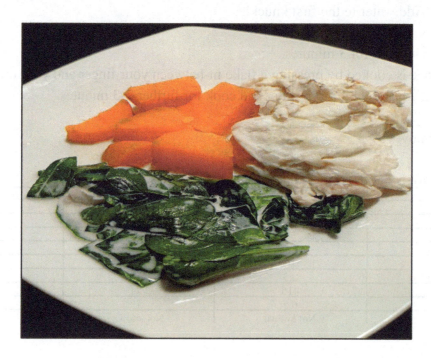

Ingredient	Quantity	Ingredient	Quantity
Fish fillet	200g or 7 oz (2 fillets)	Spinach – baby	3 cups
Garlic - crushed	4 cloves	Sweet Potato	200g or 7 oz
Onion - diced	½ medium	Coconut Cream	200ml or 7oz
Fennel seed - ground	2 Tb	Salt & Pepper to taste	
Olive Oil	3 Tb		

Method:

Heat oven to 180°C / 356°F

Infuse oil
1. In a small pot on stove, heat olive oil.
2. Add diced onion and fry till onion looks clear.
3. Add garlic and ground fennel to this.
4. Allow to fry for couple of minutes until onion turns to light brown colour.
5. Remove pot from stove, use a sieve and pour oil through this, separating onion, garlic, and fennel from infused oil.

Prepare fish dish
1. In an oven safe dish, layer fish fillet.

2. Remove stalk from baby spinach leave and discard. Add a layer baby spinach on the fish fillet.
3. Add the infused oil & salt with the coconut cream and mix through.
4. Pour the coconut cream mix on top of the fillet/baby spinach.
5. Cover the dish with aluminum foil and cook for 30 minutes to 35 minutes.
6. Take out of oven and check that the fillet is completely cooked through.
7. If cooked, then serve with the rest of the meal.
8. If fish is not cooked, put back into oven for another 10 minutes.

Boil Sweet Potato
1. Peel the skin off sweet potato.
2. Dice sweet potato into smaller pieces.
3. Place a pot of water on stove to cook sweet kumara in.
4. Add diced sweet potato and boil the water.
5. Turn down the heat, and simmer to cook the sweet potato.
6. Check to see if it is cooked.
7. If cooked, remove from stove for service.

This was a Fiji inspired meal: so **Kakana vinaka"** roughly translates to "Enjoy your food" or "Enjoy your meal.

Nutritional Analysis Per Serving

	USA	Australia	New Zealand
Energy (kJ/kcal)	1900 (454)	1827 (437)	2443 (584)
Protein (g)	24	30	31
Carbohydrate (g)	17	22	29
- Sugar (g)	4.5	7.3	13
Total Fat (g)	29	25	38
- Saturated Fat	16	11	13
Sodium (mg)	538	551	507
Dietary fiber (g)	6.4	4.6	8.9
Insoluble fiber (g)	Not known	Not known	7.5

Week 3: Day 6: Swiss Chard (Silverbeet) Lamb Lasagna

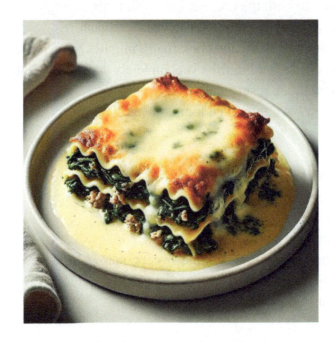

Ingredient	Quantity	Ingredient	Quantity
Garlic Infused Oil	1 Tb	Silverbeet (Swiss Chard)	8 leaves
Onion Infused Oil	1 Tb	Fresh Lasagna sheet	2 sheets
Dried Basil Leaves	1 ½ tsp	Cheese (Cheddar)	½ cup - grated
Fennel seeds	1 tsp	Milk	
Lamb Mince	200g (7 oz)	Milk	2 cups
Tomato Passata Sauce* (strained pureed tomato)	1 cup	Margarine or Butter	2 Tb
Salt & Pepper		Flour, white	

In NZ, I found a tomato passata but it still had tomato seeds in it. So, I used a sieve to remove the tomato seeds, before I used the clear passata.

Method

Turn oven to 180ºC /350ºF

Cook Lamb Mince
1. In very small pot, heat garlic infused oil and garlic infused oil.
2. While this is heating, finely grind fennel seed and dried basil leaves with mortar and pastel.
3. Add to the heated oil. Allow to fry for 30 seconds.
4. Remove from heat, use a sieve to remove the seeds and leaves from the oil. Keep the oil.

(alternatively, you can skip the above by using 2 Tb of Italian Infused Oil instead.).
5. Heat a skillet and add the sieved oil or Italian Infused Oil to this.
6. Add lamb mince and brown.
7. When mince has browned, add the tomato passata sauce. Mix well. Allow to simmer for 5 minutes, checking to make sure that the mince thickens. Turn off the heat and set aside.

Prepare Swiss Chard / Silverbeet
As discussed in an earlier section, remove the white stems from the leaves. Discard the stems. Finely chop the green leaves.

Prepare White Sauce
1. In a small pot, heat margarine or butter.
2. Add flour to this to make a paste. Cook for 1 minute.
3. Whisk in milk to this mixture to avoid forming lumps.
4. Add salt & pepper to taste.
5. Add ¾ cup of grated cheese.

Assemble Lasagna
1. Divide the lamb mince, sliced silver beet / Swiss chard and sauce into 2 lots. Lasagna sheets should be for 2 layers.
2. Using a suitable oven safe dish, at the bottom, place half of the lamb mince, then add a layer of sliced Swiss chard / Silverbeet, then layer sheets of lasagna, then add equivalent to half a cup of white sauce.
3. Repeat the same process.
4. After the final layer of lasagna sheet, add grated cheddar cheese on the top.
5. Bake for 30 minutes to 40 minutes till the lasagna is cooked.
6. Remove from oven and serve.

You can make yourself a low roughage salad to go on the side: Baby Spinach Leaves, Cucumber and Carrot with some dressing (prepare vegetables as per low roughage preparation instructions given previously).
Wishing you a tasty meal!

Nutritional Analysis Per Serving

	USA	Australia	NZ
Energy (kj/kcal)	3868 (925)	3140 (750)	3581 (856)
Protein (g)	40	45	45
Carbohydrate (g)	68	62	77
- Sugar (g)	16	14	19
Fat (g)	52	34	40.5
- Saturated Fat	19.5	13.1	16
Sodium (mg)	1490	928	1043
Dietary fiber (g)	10.7	8.7	7.4
Insoluble fiber (g)	Not known	Not known	6.4

Week 3: Day 7: Chicken Meatballs with Rice, Broccoli & Cauliflower

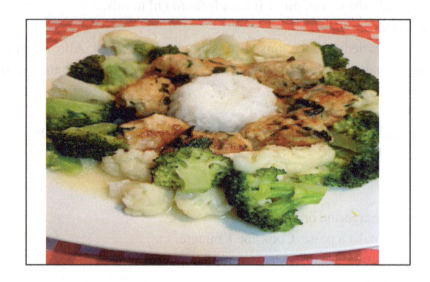

Ingredient	Quantity	Ingredient	Quantity
Garlic Infused Oil	1 Tb	Broccoli	6 florets
Onion Infused Oil	1 Tb	Salt	
Chicken - Minced	220g or 8 oz	Margarine or Butter	2 Tb
Sweet Paprika - ground	1 Tb	Milk	½ cup
Ground Cumin	1 Tb	Flour	4 Tb
Coriander - ground	1 Tb	Parsley	1 bunch
Cauliflower	6 florets	Oil for frying	
Spinach - baby	1 cup	Rice	½ cup

Method

Cook Chicken Meatballs
1. Wash minced chicken and drain.
2. Add paprika, cumin, coriander, salt, flour to the chicken and mix well.
3. Chop spinach leaves into small sizes (after taking off the stalk) add to the mixture above.
4. Add garlic infused oil and onion infused oil to this. Mix well.
5. Roll out chicken meatballs. This will make approximately 14 small meatballs.
6. Heat enough oil in a skillet and fry the meatballs, turning sides to cook all the way through.
7. Once cooked, remove from heat and put aside.

Steam or boil broccoli and cauliflower floret.
1. Prepare the broccoli and cauliflower florets as discussed in chapter 4.

2. Boil in a pot of water. Once the vegetables are cooked to your liking, drain off water and put aside.

Cook rice in the microwave
1. Put rice in microwaveable dish,
2. Wash 3 times.
3. Add 1 cup water to rice.
4. Microwave on high for 10 minutes.
5. Take out and let it sit for 3 minutes.
6. Check that the rice is cooked by pressing a flake in-between your finger and your thumb. If still uncooked, add a bit more water and cook for further 2-3 minutes.

Prepare Parsley Sauce
1. Chop parsley leaves into small pieces.
2. Add to a pot of milk and simmer for to extract flavors. Add salt to taste.
3. Take the above mix and puree through using a stick blender.
4. Sieve this through into a bowl to remove parsley leaves. Discard the leaves.
5. Heat butter/margarine to melt in a small pot.
6. Add flour to this and make a roux, using a small amount of parsley milk.
7. Add the rest of the parsley milk to this and simmer to thicken sauce.
8. Serve the above components on a plate, pouring parsley sauce on the vegetables and meatballs.

May your taste buds be delighted!

Nutritional Analysis Per Serving

	USA	Australia	NZ
Energy (kj/kcal)	2876 (687)	2458 (587)	1978 (473)
Protein (g)	53.6	46	34
Carbohydrate (g)	34	49	37
- Sugar (g)	5.9	11	10
Fat (g)	36.2	22	21
- Saturated Fat	8.8	5.5	5.3
Sodium (mg)	638	543	486
Dietary fiber (g)	5.1	6.9	3,8
Insoluble fiber (g)	Not known	Not known	2.7

SECTION 4

Country Specific, Gender Specific, Portion Guidelines To Meet Recommended Daily Allowance (USA) or Recommended Dietary Intake (Aust, NZ) For The 21 Day Low Roughage Menu (Phase 3)

Note: Gender is defined in this book as a "Male" or a "Female" for nutritional analysis as RDA / RDI and nutritional analysis programs only use these two terms for their recommendations and analysis.

United States of America Guidelines

To Meet Daily Recommended Dietary Allowance (RDA) For the 21 Days of Low Roughage Diet Menu (Phase 3)

Calculated for Average Sized Person, Undertaking light activity.

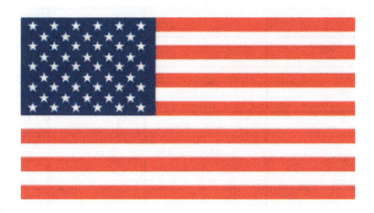

USA Female (Standard)

Age Category (years)	40-49	50-59	60-69	70-79	80 plus
Breakfast					
Porridge	1 cup	1 cup	1 cup	1 cup	1 cup
Cornflakes	1 cup	1 cup	1 cup	1 cup	1 cup
Ricies	1 cup	1 cup	1 cup	1 cup	1 cup
Stewed fruit (apple, pear, peaches)	1/3 cup	1/3 cup	1/3 cup	1/3 cup	1/3 cup
White Bread or Whole Meal Bread	2 slices	2 slices	2 slices	2 slices	2 slices
Margarine or Butter or Avocado Spread	2 teaspoons	2 teaspoons	2 teaspoons	2 teaspoons	2 teaspoons
Milk	½ cup	½ cup	½ cup	½ cup	½ cup
Fruit Juice (clear: Orange, Apple, Grapefruit)	¾ cup	¾ cup	¾ cup	¾ cup	¾ cup
Peanut Butter	2 Tb	2 Tb	2 Tb	2 Tb	2 Tb
Brown sugar	1 Tb	1 Tb	1 Tb	1 Tb	1 Tb
Morning Tea					
Water Crackers with Cream Cheese	2 crackers, 1 Tb cream cheese	2 crackers, 1 Tb cream cheese	2 crackers, 1 Tb cream cheese	2 crackers, 1 Tb cream cheese	2 crackers, 1 Tb cream cheese
Water Crackers with Cottage Cheese	2 crackers, 1 Tb cottage cheese	2 crackers, 1 Tb cottage cheese	2 crackers, 1 Tb cottage cheese	2 crackers, 1 Tb cottage cheese	2 crackers, 1 Tb cottage cheese
Water Crackers with Cheese	2 crackers, 0.7oz cheese	2 crackers, 0.7oz cheese	2 crackers, 0.7oz cheese	2 crackers, 0.7oz cheese	2 crackers, 0.7oz cheese
Arrowroot Cookies	4	2	2	2	2
Lunch					
Soup	1 cup	1 cup	1 cup	1 cup	1 cup
Protein sandwich (1 serve = 2 slices white bread/ wholemeal bread) with 20g or 0.7oz protein filling	2 serves	1 serve	1 serve	1 serve + 1 banana	2 serves
Afternoon Tea					
Water Crackers with Cream Cheese	2 crackers, 1 Tb cream cheese	2 crackers, 1 Tb cream cheese	2 crackers, 1 Tb cream cheese	2 crackers, 1 Tb cream cheese	2 crackers, 1 Tb cream cheese
Water Crackers with Cottage Cheese	2 crackers, 1 Tb cottage cheese	2 crackers, 1 Tb cottage cheese	2 crackers, 1 Tb cottage cheese	2 crackers, 1 Tb cottage cheese	2 crackers, 1 Tb cottage cheese
Water Crackers with Cheese	2 crackers, 0.7oz cheese	2 crackers, 0.7oz cheese	2 crackers, 0.7oz cheese	2 crackers, 0.7oz cheese	2 crackers, 0.7oz cheese
Fruit Flavoured Yoghurt	½ cup	½ cup	½ cup	½ cup	½ cup
Arrowroot Cookies	4	2	2	2	2
Dinner					
Protein Component	1 serve	1 serve	1 serve	1 serve	1 serve
Starch Component (potato, rice, kumara, mashed potato etc)	½ cup or 4 oz	½ cup or 4 oz	½ cup or 4 oz	½ cup or 4 oz	1/3 cup
Allowed Low Roughage Vegetables	1/3 cup	1/3 cup	1/3 cup	1/3 cup	1/3 cup
Ice Cream	½ cup	½ cup	½ cup	½ cup	½ cup
Custard	½ cup	½ cup	½ cup	½ cup	½ cup
Allowed Stewed Fruit	1/2 cup	½ cup	1/2 cup	1/2 cup	1/2 cup
Supper					
Arrowroot Cookies	4	2	2	2	2

* Milk Drink – Is required twice a day. Similarly, tea, coffees, milo and other fluid are allowed but not needed to meet the recommended daily requirement.
** once a day, ½ Cup of plain yoghurt, can be fruit flavored, no pips or seeds is recommended.

USA Male (Standard)

Age Category (years)	40-49	50-59	60-69	70-79	80 plus
Breakfast					
Porridge	1 cup	1 cup	1 cup	1 cup	1 cup
Cornflakes	1 cup	1 cup	1 cup	1 cup	1 cup
Ricies	1 cup	1 cup	1 cup	1 cup	1 cup
Stewed fruit (apple, pear, peaches)	1/3 cup	1/3 cup	1/3 cup	1/3 cup	1/3 cup
White Bread or Whole Meal Bread	2 slices	1 slice	1 slice	1 slice	1 slice
Margarine or Butter or Avocado Spread	2 teaspoons	1 teaspoon	1 teaspoon	1 teaspoon	1 teaspoon
Milk	2/3 Cup	2/3 Cup	2/3 Cup	2/3 Cup	2/3 Cup
Fruit Juice (clear: Orange, Apple, Grapefruit)	1 cup	1 cup	1 cup	1 cup	1 cup
Peanut Butter	2 Tb	2 Tb	2 Tb	2 Tb	30g
Brown sugar	2 Tb	1 Tb	1 Tb	1 Tb	1 Tb
Morning Tea					
Water Crackers with Cream Cheese: 1 serve = 2 crackers, 1 Tb cream cheese	2 serves	1 serve	1 serve	1 serve	1 serve
Water Crackers with Cottage Cheese 1 serve = 2 crackers, 1 Tb cottage cheese	2 serves	1 serve	1 serve	1 serve	1 serve
Water Crackers with Cheese 1 serve = 2 crackers, 0.7 oz cheese	2 serves	1 serve	1 serve	1 serve	1 serve
Arrowroot Cookies	4	2	2	2	2
Lunch					
Soup	1 cup	1 cup	1 cup	1 cup	1 cup
Protein sandwich (1 serve = 2 slices white bread/ wholemeal bread) with 20g or 0.7oz protein filling	2 serves	2 serves	2 serves	2 serves	2 serves
Afternoon Tea					
Water Crackers with Cream Cheese: 1 serve = 2 crackers, 1 Tb cream cheese	2 serves	1 serve	1 serve	1 serve	1 serve
Water Crackers with Cottage Cheese 1 serve = 2 crackers, 1 Tb cottage cheese	2 serves	1 serve	1 serve	1 serve	1 serve
Water Crackers with Cheese 1 serve = 2 crackers, 0.7 oz cheese	2 serves	1 serve	1 serve	1 serve	1 serve
Arrowroot Cookies	4	2	2	2	2
Soft Banana	1	1	1	1	1
With Hot chocolate	1 cup	1 cup	1 cup	1 cup	1 cup
Dinner					
Protein Component	1 serve	1 serve	1 serve	1 serve	1 serve
Starch Component (potato, rice, kumara, mashed potato etc.)	½ cup (0.4oz)	½ cup or 4 oz	½ cup	½ cup	½ cup
Allowed Low Roughage Vegetables	1/3 cup	1/3 cup	1/3 cup	1/3 cup	1/3 cup
Ice Cream	½ cup	½ cup	½ cup	½ cup	½ cup
Custard	2/3 cup	2/3 cup	2/3 cup	2/3 cup	2/3 cup
Allowed Stewed Fruit	½ cup	½ cup	½ cup	½ cup	½ cup
Supper					
Arrowroot Cookies	2	2	2	2	2
With Milky Drink	1 cup	1 cup	1 cup	1 cup	1 cup

* Milk Drink – Is required twice a day. Similarly, tea, coffees, milo and other fluid are allowed but not needed to meet the recommended daily requirement.
** once a day, ½ Cup of plain yoghurt, can be fruit flavored, no pips or seeds is recommended.

USA Female (with Diabetes)

Age Category (years)	40-49	50-59	60-69	70-79	80 plus
Breakfast					
Porridge (cooked)	1 cup	1 cup	1 cup	1 cup	1 cup
Cornflakes	1 cup	1 cup	1 cup	1 cup	1 cup
Ricies	1 cup	1 cup	1 cup	1 cup	1 cup
Stewed fruit (apple, pear, peaches) – sugar free, drained	½ cup	½ cup	1/3 cup	½ cup	½ cup
White Bread or Whole Meal Bread	2 slices	2 slices	1 slice	2 slices	2 slices
Margarine or Butter	2 teaspoons	2 teaspoons	1 teaspoon	2 teaspoons	2 teaspoons
Milk	½ cup	½ cup	½ cup	½ cup	½ cup
Low Calorie, Sugar Free Drink.	2/3 cup	2/3 cup	2/3 cup	2/3 cup	2/3 cup
Peanut Butter	2 Tb	2 Tb	2 Tb	2 Tb	2 Tb
Plain Yoghurt	½ cup	½ cup	½ cup	½ cup	½ cup
Morning Tea					
Plain Water Crackers/ Cream Cheese 1 serve= 2 crackers, 1 Tb Cream Cheese	1 serve	1 serve	1 serve	1 serve	1 serve
Plain Water Crackers/Cottage Cheese 1 serve = 2 crackers, 1 Tb cottage cheese	1 serve	1 serve	1 serve	1 serve	1 serve
Plain Water Crackers, Margarine / Tuna: 1 serve = 2 crackers, margarine, 1 Tb Tuna	1 serve	1 serve	1 serve	1 serve	1 serve
Plain Water Crackers with Cheese 1 serve = 2 crackers, 0.7oz cheese	1 serve	1 serve	1 serve	1 serve	1 serve
Digestive Biscuits	2	2	2	2	2
Milk (3.25% fat)	1 cup	1 cup	1 cup	1 cup	1 cup
Lunch					
Soup	1 cup	1 cup	1 cup	1 cup	1 cup
Protein sandwich (1 serve = 2 slices white bread/ wholemeal bread); 0.7 oz protein	2 serves	1 serve	1 serve	1 serve	1 serve
Afternoon Tea					
Plain Water Crackers/ Cream Cheese 1 serve= 2 crackers, 1 Tb Cream Cheese	1 serve	1 serve	1 serve	1 serve	1 serve
Plain Water Crackers/Cottage Cheese 1 serve = 2 crackers, 1 Tb cottage cheese	1 serve	1 serve	1 serve	1 serve	1 serve
Plain Water Crackers with Cheese 1 serve = 2 crackers, 0.7oz cheese	1 serve	1 serve	1 serve	1 serve	1 serve
Digestive Biscuits	2	2	2	2	2
Dinner					
Protein Component	1 serve	1 serve	1 serve	1 serve	1 serve
Starch Component (potato, rice, kumara, mashed potato etc.)	½ cup or 4 oz	½ cup or 4 oz	½ cup or 4 oz	½ cup or 4 oz	½ cup or 4 oz
Allowed Low Roughage Vegetables	1/3 cup	1/3 cup	1/3 cup	1/3 cup	1/3 cup
Custard – Sugar Free Or Vanilla Pudding – Sugar Free Or Chocolate Pudding – Sugar Free	½ cup	½ cup	½ cup	½ cup	½ cup
Allowed Stewed Fruit, sugar free - drained	½ cup	½ cup	½ cup	½ cup	½ cup
Sugar Free Jelly Dessert	½ cup	½ cup	½ cup	½ cup	½ cup
Supper					
Plain Water Crackers/ Cream Cheese 1 serve= 2 crackers, 1 Tb Cream Cheese	1 serve	1 serve	1 serve	1 serve	1 serve
Plain Water Crackers/Cottage Cheese 1 serve = 2 crackers, 1 Tb cottage cheese	1 serve	1 serve	1 serve	1 serve	1 serve
Plain Water Crackers with Cheese 1 serve = 2 crackers, 0.7oz cheese	1 serve	1 serve	1 serve	1 serve	1 serve
With Milk (Standard)	1 cup	2	2	2	2
Digestive Biscuits	2	1 cup	1 cup	1 cup	1 cup
** once a day, 125g or ½ Cup of plain yoghurt					

USA Male (with Diabetes)

Age Category (years)	40-49	50-59	60-69	70-79	80 plus
Breakfast					
Porridge (cooked)	1 cup	1 cup	1 cup	1 cup	1 cup
Cornflakes	1 cup	1 cup	1 cup	1 cup	1 cup
Ricies	1 cup	1 cup	1 cup	1 cup	1 cup
Stewed fruit (apple, pear, peaches) – sugar free, drained	½ cup	1/3 cup	1/3 cup	1/3 cup	1/3 cup
White Bread or Whole Meal Bread	2 slices	2 slices	1 slice	1 slice	1 slice
Margarine or Butter	2 tsp	2 tsp	1 tsp	1 tsp	1 tsp
Milk	½ cup	½ cup	½ cup	½ cup	½ cup
Low Calorie, Sugar Free Drink (Juice or Tea or Coffee etc.).	2/3 cup	2/3 cup	2/3 cup	2/3 cup	2/3 cup
Peanut Butter	2 Tb	2 Tb	2 Tb	2 Tb	2 Tb
Plain Yoghurt	½ cup	½ cup	½ cup	½ cup	½ cup
Morning Tea					
Plain Water Crackers with Cream Cheese: 1 serve = 2 crackers, 1 Tb cream cheese	2 serves	2 serves	1 serve	1 serve	1 serve
Plain Water Crackers with Cottage Cheese : 1 serve = 2 crackers, 1 Tb cottage cheese	2 serves	2 serves	1 serve	1 serve	1 serve
Plain Water Crackers, Margarine with Tuna 1 serve = 2 crackers, 1 tsp margarine, 1 Tb Tuna	2 serves	2 serves	1 serve	1 serve	1 serve
Plain Water Crackers with Cheese: 1 serve = 2 crackers, 0.7oz cheese	2 serves	2 serves	1 serve	1 serve	1 serve
Digestive Biscuits With	4	4	2	2	2
Milk (3.25% fat)	1 cup	1 cup	1 cup	1 cup	1 cup
Lunch					
Soup	1 cup	1 cup	1 cup	1 cup	1 cup
Protein sandwich (1 serve = 2 slices white bread/ wholemeal bread) with 20g or 0.7 oz protein filling	2 serves	2 serves	2 serves	2 serve	2 serves
Afternoon Tea					
Water Crackers with Cream Cheese: 1 serve = 2 crackers, 1 Tb cream cheese	2 serves	2 serves	2 serves	1 serve	1 serve
Plain Water Crackers with Cottage Cheese : 1 serve = 2 crackers, 1 Tb cottage cheese	2 serves	2 serves	2 serves	1 serve	1 serve
Plain Water Crackers with Cheese: 1 serve = 2 crackers, 0.7oz cheese	2 serves	2 serves	2 serves	1 serve	1 serve
Digestive Biscuits	4	4	4	2	2
Dinner					
Protein Component	1 serve	1 serve	1 serve	1 serve	1 serve
Starch Component (potato, rice, kumara, mashed potato etc.)	½ cup or 4 oz	½ cup or 4 oz	½ cup or 4 oz	½ cup or 4 oz	½ cup or 4 oz
Allowed Low Roughage Vegetables	1/3 cup	1/3 cup	1/3 cup	1/3 cup	1/3 cup
Custard – Sugar Free Or Vanilla Pudding – Sugar Free Or Chocolate Pudding – Sugar Free	½ cup	½ cup	½ cup	½ cup	½ cup
Allowed Stewed Fruit, sugar free - drained	½ cup	½ cup	½ cup	½ cup	½ cup
Sugar Free Jelly Dessert	½ cup	½ cup	½ cup	½ cup	½ cup
Supper					
Water Crackers with Cream Cheese: 1 serve = 2 crackers, 1 Tb cream cheese	2 serves	2 serves	2 serves	1 serve	1 serve
Plain Water Crackers with Cottage Cheese : 1 serve = 2 crackers, 1 Tb cottage cheese	2 serves	2 serves	2 serves	1 serve	1 serve
Plain Water Crackers with Cheese: 1 serve = 2 crackers, 0.7oz cheese	2 serves	2 serves	2 serves	1 serve	1 serve
With Milk (Standard)	1 cup	1 cup	1 cup	1 cup	1 cup
Digestive Biscuits	4	4	4	2	2
** once a day, 125g or ½ Cup of plain yoghurt					

New Zealand Guidelines

To Meet Daily Recommended Dietary Intake (RDI) For The 21 Days of Low Roughage Diet Menu (Phase 3)

Calculated for Average Sized Person, Undertaking light activity.

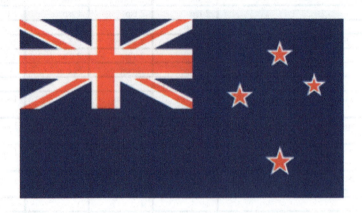

NZ Female (Standard)

Age Category	40 – 49	50 – 59	60 – 69	70 – 79	80+
Breakfast					
Porridge	1 cup	1 cup	1 cup	1 cup	1 cup
Cornflakes	1 cup	1 cup	1 cup	1 cup	1 cup
Rice bubbles	1 cup	1 cup	1 cup	1 cup	1 cup
Stewed fruit (apple, pear, peaches)	1/3 cup	1/3 cup	1/3 cup	1/3 cup	1/3 cup
White Bread or Whole Meal Bread	2 slices	2 slices	2 slice	2 slice	2 slice
Plant Based Spread, Butter or Avocado Spread	2 tsp	2 tsp	2 tsp	2 tsp	2 tsp
Milk	½ cup	½ cup	½ cup	½ cup	½ cup
Fruit Juice (clear: Orange, Apple, Grapefruit)	¾ cup	¾ cup	¾ cup	¾ cup	¾ cup
Peanut Butter	2 Tb	2 Tb	2 Tb	2 Tb	2 Tb
Brown sugar	1 Tb	1 Tb	1 Tb	1 Tb	1 Tb
Morning Tea					
Water Crackers with Cream Cheese: 1 serve = 2 crackers, 1 Tb cream cheese	1 serve	1 serve	1 serve	1 serve	1 serve
Water Crackers with Cottage Cheese: 1 serve = 2 crackers, 1 Tb cottage cheese	1 serve	1 serve	1 serve	1 serve	1 serve
Water Crackers with Cheese: 1 serve = 2 crackers, 20g cheese	1 serve	1 serve	1 serve	1 serve	1 serve
Arrowroot Cookies	4	2	2	2	2
Lunch					
Soup	1 cup	1 cup	1 cup	1 cup	1 cup
Protein sandwich (1 serve = 2 slices white bread/ wholemeal bread) with 20g protein filling	2 serves	1 serve	1 serve	1 serve	1 serve
Banana	1 medium	1 medium	1 medium	1 medium	1 medium
Afternoon Tea					
Water Crackers with Cream Cheese: 1 serve = 2 crackers, 1 Tb cream cheese	1 serve	1 serve	1 serve	1 serve	1 serve
Water Crackers with Cottage Cheese: 1 serve = 2 crackers, 1 Tb cottage cheese	1 serve	1 serve	1 serve	1 serve	1 serve
Water Crackers with Cheese: 1 serve = 2 crackers, 20g cheese	1 serve	1 serve	1 serve	1 serve	1 serve
Fruit Flavored Yoghurt	½ cup	½ cup	½ cup	½ cup	½ cup
Arrowroot Cookies	4	2	2	2	2
Dinner					
Protein Component	1 serve	1 serve	1 serve	1 serve	1 serve
Starch Component (potato, rice, kumara, mashed potato etc.)	½ cup	½ cup	½ cup	½ cup	½ cup
Allowed Low Roughage Vegetables	1/3 cup	1/3 cup	1/3 cup	1/3 cup	1/3 cup
Ice Cream	½ cup	½ cup	½ cup	½ cup	½ cup
Custard	½ cup	½ cup	½ cup	½ cup	½ cup
Allowed Stewed Fruit	1/2 cup	1/2 cup	1/2 cup	1/2 cup	1/2 cup
Supper					
Arrowroot Cookies	4	2	2	2	2

* Milk Drink – Is required twice a day. Similarly, tea, coffees, milo and other fluid are allowed but not needed to meet the recommended daily requirement.
** once a day, ½ Cup of plain yoghurt, can be fruit flavored, no pips or seeds is recommended

NZ Male (Standard)

Age Category	40 – 49	50 – 59	60 – 69	70 – 79	80+
Breakfast					
Porridge	1 cup	1 cup	1 cup	1 cup	1 cup
Cornflakes	1 cup	1 cup	1 cup	1 cup	1 cup
Rice bubbles	1 cup	1 cup	1 cup	1 cup	1 cup
Stewed fruit (apple, pear, peaches)	1/3 cup	1/3 cup	1/3 cup	1/3 cup	1/3 cup
White Bread or Whole Meal Bread	2 slices	1 slice	1 slice	1 slice	1 slice
Plant Based Spread, Butter or Avocado Spread	2 teaspoons	1 teaspoon	1 teaspoon	1 teaspoon	1 teaspoon
Milk	2/3 Cup	2/3 Cup	2/3 Cup	2/3 Cup	2/3 Cup
Fruit Juice (clear: Orange, Apple, Grapefruit)	1 cup	1 cup	1 cup	1 cup	1 cup
Peanut Butter	2 Tb	2 Tb	2 Tb	2 Tb	2 Tb
Brown sugar	2 Tb	1 Tb	1 Tb	1 Tb	1 Tb
Morning Tea					
Water Crackers with Cream Cheese: 1 serve = 2 crackers, 1 Tb cream cheese	1 serve	1 serve	1 serve	1 serve	1 serve
Water Crackers with Cottage Cheese: 1 serve = 2 crackers, 1 Tb cottage cheese	1 serve	1 serve	1 serve	1 serve	1 serve
Water Crackers with Cheese: 1 serve = 2 crackers, 20g cheese	1 serve	1 serve	1 serve	1 serve	1 serve
Arrowroot Cookies	4	2	2	2	2
Lunch					
Soup	1 cup	1 cup	1 cup	1 cup	1 cup
Protein sandwich (1 serve = 2 slices white bread/ wholemeal bread) with 20g protein filling	2 serves	2 serves	2 serves	2 serves	2 serves
Afternoon Tea					
Water Crackers with Cream Cheese: 1 serve = 2 crackers, 1 Tb cream cheese	1 serve	1 serve	1 serve	1 serve	1 serve
Water Crackers with Cottage Cheese: 1 serve = 2 crackers, 1 Tb cottage cheese	1 serve	1 serve	1 serve	1 serve	1 serve
Water Crackers with Cheese: 1 serve = 2 crackers, 20g cheese	1 serve	1 serve	1 serve	1 serve	1 serve
Arrowroot Cookies	4	2	2	½ cup	2
Soft Banana	1	1	1	2	1
With Hot chocolate	1 cup	1 cup	1 cup	1 cup	1 cup
Dinner					
Protein Component	1 serve	1 serve	1 serve	1 serve	1 serve
Starch Component (potato, rice, kumara, mashed potato etc.)	½ cup	½ cup	½ cup	½ cup	½ cup
Allowed Low Roughage Vegetables	1/3 cup	1/3 cup	1/3 cup	1/3 cup	1/3 cup
Ice Cream	½ cup	½ cup	½ cup	½ cup	½ cup
Custard	2/3 cup	2/3 cup	2/3 cup	2/3 cup	½ cup
Allowed Stewed Fruit	½ cup	½ cup	½ cup	½ cup	1/2 cup
Supper					
Arrowroot Cookies	2	2	2	2	2
With Milky Drink	1 cup	1 cup	1 cup	1 cup	1 cup

* Milky Drink – Is required twice a day. Similarly, tea, coffees, milo and other fluid are allowed but not needed to meet the recommended daily requirement.
** once a day, ½ cup of plain yoghurt, can be fruit flavored, no pips or seeds is recommended.

NZ Female (with Diabetes)

Age Category	40 – 49	50 – 59	60 – 69	70 – 79	80 +
Breakfast					
Porridge (cooked)	1 cup	1 cup	1 cup	1 cup	1 cup
Cornflakes	1 cup	1 cup	1 cup	1 cup	1 cup
Rice bubbles	1 cup	1 cup	1 cup	1 cup	1 cup
Stewed fruit (apple, pear, peaches) – sugar free, drained	½ cup	½ cup	1/3 cup	½ cup	½ cup
White Bread or Whole Meal Bread	2 slices	2 slices	1 slices	2 slices	2 slices
Plant Based Spread, Butter or Avocado Spread	2 tsp	2 tsp	1 tsp	2 tsp	2 tsp
Milk	½ cup	½ cup	½ cup	½ cup	½ cup
Low Calorie, Sugar Free Drink (Juice or Tea or Coffee etc.).	2/3 cup	2/3 cup	2/3 cup	2/3 cup	2/3 cup
Peanut Butter	2 Tb	2 Tb	2 Tb	2 Tb	2 Tb
Plain Yoghurt	½ cup	½ cup	½ cup	½ cup	½ cup
Morning Tea					
Plain Water Crackers with Cream Cheese: 1 serve = 2 crackers, 1 Tb cream cheese	1 serve	1 serve	1 serve	1 serve	1 serve
Plain Water Crackers with Cottage Cheese: 1 serve = 2 crackers, 1 Tb cottage cheese	1 serve	1 serve	1 serve	1 serve	1 serve
Plain Water Crackers, with Tuna: 1 serve = 2 crackers, 1 Tb Tuna	1 serve	1 serve	1 serve	1 serve	1 serve
Plain Water Crackers with Cheese: 1 serve = 2 crackers, 20 g Cheese	1 serve	1 serve	1 serve	1 serve	1 serve
Digestive Biscuits With	2	2	2	2	2
Milk (3.25% fat)	1 cup	1 cup	1 cup	1 cup	1 cup
Lunch					
Soup	1 cup	1 cup	1 cup	1 cup	1 cup
Protein sandwich (1 serve = 2 slices white bread/ wholemeal bread) with 30g protein filling	2 serves	1 serve	1 serve	1 serve	1 serve
Afternoon Tea					
Plain Water Crackers with Cream Cheese: 1 serve = 2 crackers, 1 Tb cream cheese	1 serve	1 serve	1 serve	1 serve	1 serve
Plain Water Crackers with Cottage Cheese: 1 serve = 2 crackers, 1 Tb cottage cheese	1 serve	1 serve	1 serve	1 serve	1 serve
Plain Water Crackers, with Tuna: 1 serve = 2 crackers, 1 Tb Tuna	1 serve	1 serve	1 serve	1 serve	1 serve
Digestive Biscuits	2	2	2	2	2
Dinner					
Protein Component	1 serve	1 serve	1 serve	1 serve	1 serve
Starch Component (potato, rice, kumara, mashed potato etc.)	½ cup	½ cup	½ cup	½ cup	½ cup
Allowed Low Roughage Vegetables	1/3 cup	1/3 cup	1/3 cup	1/3 cup	1/3 cup
Custard – Sugar Free Or Vanilla Pudding – Sugar Free Or Chocolate Pudding – Sugar Free	½ cup	½ cup	½ cup	½ cup	½ cup
Allowed Stewed Fruit, sugar free – drained	½ cup	½ cup	½ cup	½ cup	½ cup
Sugar Free Jelly Dessert	½ cup	½ cup	½ cup	½ cup	½ cup
Supper					
Plain Water Crackers with Cream Cheese: 1 serve = 2 crackers, 1 Tb cream cheese	1 serve	1 serve	1 serve	1 serve	1 serve
Plain Water Crackers with Cottage Cheese: 1 serve = 2 crackers, 1 Tb cottage cheese	1 serve	1 serve	1 serve	1 serve	1 serve
Plain Water Crackers with Cheese: 1 serve = 2 crackers, 20 g Cheese	1 serve	1 serve	1 serve	1 serve	1 serve
With Milk (Standard)	1 cup	2	2	2	2
Digestive Biscuits	2	1 cup	1 cup	1	1 cup
* Once a day, 125g or ½ Cup of plain yoghurt					

NZ Male (with Diabetes)

Age Category	40-49	50 – 59	60 – 69	70 – 79	80+
Breakfast					
Porridge	1 cup	1 cup	1 cup	1 cup	1 cup
Cornflakes	1 cup	1 cup	1 cup	1 cup	1 cup
Rice bubbles	1 cup	1 cup	1 cup	1 cup	1 cup
Stewed fruit (apple, pear, peaches) – sugar free, drained	½ cup	1/3 cup	1/3 cup	1/3 cup	1/3 cup
White Bread or Whole Meal Bread	2 slices	2 slices	1 slice	1 slice	1 slice
Plant Based Spread, Butter or Avocado Spread	2 teaspoons	2 teaspoons	1 teaspoon	1 teaspoon	1 teaspoon
Milk	½ cup	½ cup	½ cup	½ cup	½ cup
Low Calorie, Sugar Free Drink (Juice or Tea or Coffee etc).	2/3 cup	2/3 cup	2/3 cup	2/3 cup	2/3 cup
Peanut Butter	2 Tb	2 Tb	2 Tb	2 Tb	2 Tb
Plain Yoghurt	½ cup	½ cup	½ cup	½ cup	½ cup
Morning Tea					
Plain Water Crackers with Cream Cheese: 1 serve = 2 crackers, 1 Tb cream cheese	1 serve	1 serve	1 serve	1 serve	1 serve
Plain Water Crackers with Cottage Cheese: 1 serve = 2 crackers, 1 Tb cottage cheese	1 serve	1 serve	1 serve	1 serve	1 serve
Plain Water Crackers, with Tuna: 1 serve = 2 crackers, 1 Tb Tuna	1 serve	1 serve	1 serve	1 serve	1 serve
Plain Water Crackers with Cheese: 1 serve = 2 crackers, 20 g Cheese	1 serve	1 serve	1 serve	1 serve	1 serve
Digestive Biscuits	4	4	2	2	2
With Milk (3.25% fat)	1 cup	1 cup	1 cup	1 cup	1 cup
Lunch					
Soup	1 cup	1 cup	1 cup	1 cup	1 cup
Protein sandwich (1 serve = 2 slices white bread/ wholemeal bread) with 1 oz protein filling	2 serves	2 serves	2 serves	2 serves	2 serves
Afternoon Tea					
Plain Water Crackers with Cream Cheese: 1 serve = 2 crackers, 1 Tb cream cheese	1 serve	1 serve	1 serve	1 serve	1 serve
Plain Water Crackers with Cottage Cheese: 1 serve = 2 crackers, 1 Tb cottage cheese	1 serve	1 serve	1 serve	1 serve	1 serve
Plain Water Crackers with Cheese: 1 serve = 2 crackers, 20 g Cheese	1 serve	1 serve	1 serve	1 serve	1 serve
Digestive Biscuits	4	4	4	2	2
Dinner					
Protein Component	1 serve	1 serve	1 serve	1 serve	1 serve
Starch Component (potato, rice, kumara, mashed potato etc.)	½ cup	½ cup	½ cup	½ cup	½ cup
Allowed Low Roughage Vegetables	1/3 cup	1/3 cup	1/3 cup	1/3 cup	1/3 cup
Custard – Sugar Free or Vanilla Pudding – Sugar Free or Sugar Free Chocolate Pudding	½ cup	½ cup	½ cup	½ cup	½ cup
Allowed Stewed Fruit, sugar free – drained	½ cup	½ cup	½ cup	½ cup	½ cup
Sugar Free Jelly	½ cup	½ cup	½ cup	½ cup	½ cup
Supper					
Plain Water Crackers with Cream Cheese: 1 serve = 2 crackers, 1 Tb cream cheese	1 serve	1 serve	1 serve	1 serve	1 serve
Plain Water Crackers with Cottage Cheese: 1 serve = 2 crackers, 1 Tb cottage cheese	1 serve	1 serve	1 serve	1 serve	1 serve
Plain Water Crackers with Cheese: 1 serve = 2 crackers, 20 g Cheese	1 serve	1 serve	1 serve	1 serve	1 serve
With Milk (3.25% fat)	1 cup	1 cup	1 cup	1 cup	1 cup
Digestive Biscuits	4	4	4	2	2

*Once a day, 125g of plain yoghurt

Australian Guidelines

To Meet Daily Recommended Dietary Intake For The 21 Day Low Roughage Diet Menu (Phase 3)

Calculated for Average Sized Person, Undertaking light activity.

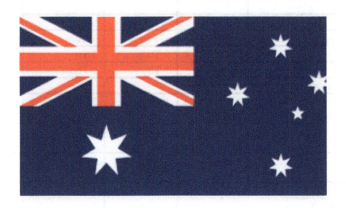

Australian Female (Standard)

Age Categories	40 – 49	50 – 59	60 – 69	70 -79	80 +
Breakfast					
Porridge	1 cup	1 cup	1 cup	1 cup	1 cup
Cornflakes	1 cup	1 cup	1 cup	1 cup	1 cup
Ricies	1 cup	1 cup	1 cup	1 cup	1 cup
Stewed fruit (apple, pear, peaches)	1/3 cup	1/3 cup	1/3 cup	1/3 cup	1/3 cup
White Bread or Whole Meal Bread	2 slices	2 slices	2 slices	2 slices	2 slice
Plant Based Spread, Butter or Avocado Spread	2 teaspoons	2 teaspoons	2 teaspoons	2 teaspoons	2 teaspoons
Milk	½ cup	½ cup	½ cup	½ cup	½ cup
Fruit Juice (clear: Orange, Apple, Grapefruit)	¾ cup	¾ cup	¾ cup	¾ cup	¾ cup
Peanut Butter	2 Tb	2 Tb	2 Tb	2 Tb	2 Tb
Brown sugar	1 Tb	1 Tb	1 Tb	1 Tb	1 Tb
Morning Tea					
Water Crackers with Cream Cheese: 1 serve = 2 crackers, 1 Tb cream cheese	1 serve	1 serve	1 serve	1 serve	1 serve
Water Crackers with Cottage Cheese: 1 serve = 2 crackers, 1 Tb cottage cheese	1 serve	1 serve	1 serve	1 serve	1 serve
Water Crackers with Cheese: 1 serve = 2 crackers, 20g cheese	1 serve	1 serve	1 serve	1 serve	1 serve
Arrowroot Cookies	4	2	2	2	2
Lunch					
Soup	1 cup	1 cup	1 cup	1 cup	1 cup
Protein sandwich (1 serve = 2 slices white bread/ wholemeal bread) with 20g protein filling	2 serves	1 serve	1 serve	1 serve	1 serve
Banana	1 medium	1 medium	1 medium	1 medium	1 medium
Afternoon Tea					
Water Crackers with Cream Cheese: 1 serve = 2 crackers, 1 Tb cream cheese	1 serve	1 serve	1 serve	1 serve	1 serve
Water Crackers with Cottage Cheese: 1 serve = 2 crackers, 1 Tb cottage cheese	1 serve	1 serve	1 serve	1 serve	1 serve
Water Crackers with Cheese: 1 serve = 2 crackers, 20g cheese	1 serve	1 serve	1 serve	1 serve	1 serve
Fruit Flavored Yoghurt	½ cup	½ cup	½ cup	½ cup	½ cup
Arrowroot Cookies	4	2	2	2	2
Dinner					
Protein Component	1 serve	1 serve	1 serve	1 serve	1 serve
Starch Component (potato, rice, kumara, mashed potato etc.)	½ cup	½ cup	½ cup	½ cup	½ cup
Allowed Low Roughage Vegetables	1/3 cup	1/3 cup	1/3 cup	1/3 cup	1/3 cup
Ice Cream	½ cup	½ cup	½ cup	½ cup	½ cup
Custard	½ cup	½ cup	½ cup	½ cup	½ cup
Allowed Stewed Fruit	1/2 cup	1/2 cup	1/2 cup	1/2 cup	1/2 cup
Supper					
Arrowroot Cookies	4	2	2	2	2

* Milk Drink – Is required twice a day. Similarly, tea, coffees, milo and other fluid are allowed but not needed to meet the recommended daily requirement.
** Once a day, ½ Cup of plain yoghurt, can be fruit flavored, no pips or seeds is recommended.

Australian Male (Standard)

Age Category	40-49	50-59	60-69	70-79	80+
Breakfast					
Porridge	1 cup	1 cup	1 cup	1 cup	1 cup
Cornflakes	1 cup	1 cup	1 cup	1 cup	1 cup
Ricies	1 cup	1 cup	1 cup	1 cup	1 cup
Stewed fruit (apple, pear, peaches)	1/3 cup	1/3 cup	80g	1/3 cup	1/3 cup
White Bread or Whole Meal Bread	2 slices	1 slice	1 slice	1 slice	1 slice
Plant Based Spread, Butter or Avocado Spread	2 teaspoons	1 teaspoon	1 teaspoon	1 teaspoon	1 teaspoon
Milk or Plain or Fruit Flavored Yoghurt	2/3 Cup	2/3 Cup	2/3 Cup	2/3 Cup	2/3 Cup
Fruit Juice (clear: Orange, Apple, Grapefruit)	1 cup	1 cup	1 cup	1 cup	1 cup
Cream	2 Tb	2 Tb	30g	2 Tb	30g
Peanut Butter	2 Tb	1 Tb	1 Tb	1 Tb	1 Tb
Morning Tea					
Water Crackers with Cream Cheese: 1 serve = 2 crackers, 1 Tb cream cheese	1 serve	1 serve	1 serve	1 serve	1 serve
Water Crackers with Cottage Cheese: 1 serve = 2 crackers, 1 Tb cottage cheese	1 serve	1 serve	1 serve	1 serve	1 serve
Water Crackers with Cheese: 1 serve = 2 crackers, 20g cheese	1 serve	1 serve	1 serve	1 serve	1 serve
Arrowroot Cookies	4	2	2	2	2
Lunch					
Soup	1 cup	1 cup	1 cup	1 cup	1 cup
Protein sandwich (1 serve = 2 slices white bread/ wholemeal bread) with 20g protein filling	2 serves	2 serves	2 serves	2 serves	2 serves
Age Categories	40-49	50-59	60-69	70-79	80+
Afternoon Tea					
Water Crackers with Cream Cheese: 1 serve = 2 crackers, 1 Tb cream cheese	1 serve	1 serve	1 serve	1 serve	1 serve
Water Crackers with Cottage Cheese: 1 serve = 2 crackers, 1 Tb cottage cheese	1 serve	1 serve	1 serve	1 serve	1 serve
Water Crackers with Cheese: 1 serve = 2 crackers, 20g cheese	1 serve	1 serve	1 serve	1 serve	1 serve
Arrowroot Cookies	4	2	2	2	2
Soft Banana	1	1	1	1	1
With Hot chocolate	1 cup	1 cup	1 cup	1 cup	1 cup
Dinner					
Protein Component	1 serve	1 serve	1 serve	1 serve	1 serve
Starch Component (potato, rice, kumara, mashed potato etc.)	½ cup	½ cup	½ cup	½ cup	½ cup
Allowed Low Roughage Vegetables	1/3 cup	1/3 cup	1/3 cup	1/3 cup	1/3 cup
Ice Cream	½ cup	½ cup	½ cup	½ cup	½ cup
Custard	2/3 cup	2/3 cup	2/3 cup	2/3 cup	2/3 cup
Allowed Stewed Fruit	½ cup	½ cup	½ cup	½ cup	½ cup
Supper					
Arrowroot Cookies	2	2	2	2	2
With Milky Drink	1 cup	1 cup	1 cup	1 cup	1 cup

* Milky Drink – Is required twice a day. Similarly, tea, coffees, milo and other fluid are allowed but not needed to meet the recommended daily requirement.

** Once a day, ½ cup of plain yoghurt, can be fruit flavored, no pips or seeds is recommended.

Australian Female (with Diabetes)

Age Categories	40 – 49	50 – 59	60 – 69	70 – 79	80 +
Breakfast					
Porridge (cooked)	1 cup	1 cup	1 cup	1 cup	1 cup
Cornflakes	1 cup	1 cup	1 cup	1 cup	1 cup
Ricies	1 cup	1 cup	1 cup	1 cup	1 cup
Stewed fruit (apple, pear, peaches) – sugar free, drained	½ cup	½ cup	1/3 cup	½ cup	½ cup
White Bread or Whole Meal Bread	2 slices	2 slices	1 slices	2 slices	2 slices
Margarine, Butter or Avocado Spread	2 tsp	2 tsp	2 tsp	2 tsp	2 tsp
Milk	½ cup	½ cup	½ cup	½ cup	½ cup
Low Calorie, Sugar Free Drink (Juice or Tea or Coffee etc.).	2/3 cup	2/3 cup	2/3 cup	2/3 cup	2/3 cup
Peanut Butter	2 Tb	2 Tb	2 Tb	2 Tb	2 Tb
Plain Yoghurt	½ cup	½ cup	½ cup	½ cup	½ cup
Morning Tea					
Plain Water Crackers with Cream Cheese: 1 serve = 2 crackers, 1 Tb cream cheese	1 serve	1 serve	1 serve	1 serve	1 serve
Plain Water Crackers with Cottage Cheese: 1 serve = 2 crackers, 1 Tb cottage cheese	1 serve	1 serve	1 serve	1 serve	1 serve
Plain Water Crackers, with Tuna: 1 serve = 2 crackers, 1 Tb Tuna	1 serve	1 serve	1 serve	1 serve	1 serve
Plain Water Crackers with Cheese: 1 serve = 2 crackers, 20g cheese	1 serve	1 serve	1 serve	1 serve	1 serve
Digestive Biscuits With	2	2	2	2	2
Milk (3.25% fat)	1 cup	1 cup	1 cup	1 cup	1 cup
Lunch					
Soup	1 cup	1 cup	1 cup	1 cup	1 cup
Protein sandwich (1 serve = 2 slices white bread/ wholemeal bread) with 20g protein filling	2 serves	1 serve	1 serve	1 serve	1 serve
Afternoon Tea					
Plain Water Crackers with Cream Cheese: 1 serve = 2 crackers, 1 Tb cream cheese	1 serve	1 serve	1 serve	1 serve	1 serve
Plain Water Crackers with Cottage Cheese: 1 serve = 2 crackers, 1 Tb cottage cheese	1 serve	1 serve	1 serve	1 serve	1 serve
Plain Water Crackers with Cheese: 1 serve = 2 crackers, 20g cheese	1 serve	1 serve	1 serve	1 serve	1 serve
Digestive Biscuits	2	2	2	2	2
Dinner					
Protein Component	1 serve	1 serve	1 serve	1 serve	1 serve
Starch Component (potato, rice, kumara, mashed potato etc.)	½ cup	½ cup	½ cup	½ cup	½ cup
Allowed Low Roughage Vegetables	1/3 cup	1/3 cup	1/3 cup	1/3 cup	1/3 cup
Custard – Sugar Free Or Vanilla Pudding – Sugar Free Or Chocolate Pudding – Sugar Free	½ cup	½ cup	½ cup	½ cup	½ cup
Allowed Stewed Fruit, sugar free - drained	½ cup	½ cup	½ cup	½ cup	½ cup
Sugar Free Jelly Dessert	½ cup	½ cup	½ cup	½ cup	½ cup
Supper					
Plain Water Crackers with Cream Cheese: 1 serve = 2 crackers, 1 Tb cream cheese	1 serve	1 serve	1 serve	1 serve	1 serve
Plain Water Crackers with Cottage Cheese: 1 serve = 2 crackers, 1 Tb cottage cheese	1 serve	1 serve	1 serve	1 serve	1 serve
Plain Water Crackers with Cheese: 1 serve = 2 crackers, 20g cheese	1 serve	1 serve	1 serve	1 serve	1 serve
With Milk (Standard)	1 cup	2	2	2	2
Digestive Biscuits	2	1 cup	1 cup	1 cup	1 cup (250g)

* Once a day, 125g or ½ Cup of plain yoghurt

Australian Male (with Diabetes)

Age Categories	40 – 49	50 – 59	60 – 69	70 – 79	80 +
Breakfast					
Porridge	1 cup	1 cup	1 cup	1 cup	1 cup
Cornflakes	1 cup	1 cup	1 cup	1 cup	1 cup
Ricies	1 cup	1 cup	1 cup	1 cup	1 cup
Stewed fruit (apple, pear, peaches) – sugar free, drained	½ cup	1/3 cup	1/3 cup	1/3 cup	1/3 cup
White Bread or Whole Meal Bread	2 slices	2 slices	1 slice	1 slice	1 slice
Margarine or Butter or Avocado Spread	2 teaspoons	2 teaspoons	1 teaspoon	1 teaspoon	1 teaspoon
Milk	½ cup	½ cup	½ cup	½ cup	½ cup
Low Calorie, Sugar Free Drink (Juice or Tea or Coffee etc.).	2/3 cup	2/3 cup	2/3 cup	2/3 cup	2/3 cup
Peanut Butter	2 Tb	2 Tb	2 Tb	2 Tb	2 Tb
Plain Yoghurt	½ cup	½ cup	½ cup	½ cup	½ cup
Morning Tea					
Plain Water Crackers with Cream Cheese: 1 serve = 2 crackers, 1 Tb cream cheese	1 serve	1 serve	1 serve	1 serve	1 serve
Plain Water Crackers with Cottage Cheese: 1 serve = 2 crackers, 1 Tb cottage cheese	1 serve	1 serve	1 serve	1 serve	1 serve
Plain Water Crackers, with Tuna: 1 serve = 2 crackers, 1 Tb Tuna	1 serve	1 serve	1 serve	1 serve	1 serve
Plain Water Crackers with Cheese: 1 serve = 2 crackers, 20g cheese	1 serve	1 serve	1 serve	1 serve	1 serve
Digestive Biscuits	4	4	2	2	2
With Milk (3.25% fat)	1 cup	1 cup	1 cup	1 cup	1 cup
Lunch					
Soup	1 cup	1 cup	1 cup	1 cup	1 cup
Protein sandwich (1 serve = 2 slices white bread/ wholemeal bread) with 20g protein filling	2 serves	2 serves	2 serves	2 serves	2 serves
Afternoon Tea					
Plain Water Crackers with Cream Cheese: 1 serve = 2 crackers, 1 Tb cream cheese	1 serve	1 serve	1 serve	1 serve	1 serve
Plain Water Crackers with Cottage Cheese: 1 serve = 2 crackers, 1 Tb cottage cheese	1 serve	1 serve	1 serve	1 serve	1 serve
Plain Water Crackers with Cheese: 1 serve = 2 crackers, 20g cheese	1 serve	1 serve	1 serve	1 serve	1 serve
Digestive Biscuits	4	4	4		2
Dinner					
Protein Component	1 serve	1 serve	1 serve	1 serve	1 serve
Starch Component (potato, rice, kumara, mashed potato etc)	½ cup	½ cup	½ cup	½ cup	½ cup
Allowed Low Roughage Vegetables	1/3 cup	1/3 cup	1/3 cup	1/3 cup	1/3 cup
Custard – Sugar Free or Vanilla Pudding – Sugar Free or Sugar Free Chocolate Pudding	½ cup	½ cup	½ cup	½ cup	½ cup
Allowed Stewed Fruit, sugar free – drained	½ cup	½ cup	½ cup	½ cup	½ cup
Sugar Free Jelly	½ cup	½ cup	½ cup	½ cup	½ cup
Supper					
Plain Water Crackers with Cream Cheese: 1 serve = 2 crackers, 1 Tb cream cheese	1 serve	1 serve	1 serve	1 serve	1 serve
Plain Water Crackers with Cottage Cheese: 1 serve = 2 crackers, 1 Tb cottage cheese	1 serve	1 serve	1 serve	1 serve	1 serve
Plain Water Crackers with Cheese: 1 serve = 2 crackers, 20g cheese	1 serve	1 serve	1 serve	1 serve	1 serve
With Milk (3.25% fat)	1 cup	1 cup	1 cup	1 cup	1 cup
Digestive Biscuits	4	4	4	2	2
** once a day, 125g of plain yoghurt					

Feedback

"If you enjoyed this book, I'd be incredibly grateful if you could take a moment to leave a review. Your feedback helps other readers discover this story and supports my work as an author. Also, if you have suggestions on how to improve this book or possible topics to include in this book, please share your thoughts by clicking on the link below:

https://maximisednutrition.com/lwd_feedback/

This book is part of a series of books called, "Empower Series". The aim of this series is to empower you with both knowledge and practical information in holistic health so that you can live the best life you can.

Thank you,

Prem Nand, Clinical Dietitian – Nutritionist, NZRD.

Legal Disclaimer

This book provides helpful dietary advice for managing Diverticulitis and Diverticular Disease. It has been created by Maximised Nutrition Ltd (maximisednutrition.com).

By using this guide, you agree to the following terms. If you do not agree, please avoid using the content.

We have done our best to offer practical tips, but please remember, this information is not a substitute for personalized advice from a qualified healthcare professional. The author, a Registered Dietitian based in New Zealand, is also allowed to practice in Australia, but not in other countries, like the USA. So, if you are outside of these areas, consider this guide more of a general resource.

It is important to note that this book is not meant to replace medical care, and you should see a doctor if your symptoms do not improve. The information here is accurate as of the time it was written, but it might not cover every detail.

By using this book, you agree not to hold Prem Nand, Clinical Dietitian-Nutritionist, Maximised Nutrition Ltd, or any of its owners, agents, or employees responsible for any issues that come up from using this information, unless there has been gross negligence or intentional harm.

.If you have concerns about the content of this educational product, please send an e-mail (**publisher@maximisednutrition.com**) or write us at the following address:

Maximised Nutrition Limited
C/- Whangarei Wellness Centre, Level 1
25 Rathbone Street
Whangarei 0110, New Zealand

Made in the USA
Monee, IL
09 December 2024